MW00961928

Lewy Body Dementia:

Causes, Tests and Treatment Options

Adam Wainwright, MA, Erik Stevenson MD (Ed.)

© 2012 Adam Wainwright, MA, Erik Stevenson MD

All Rights Reserved worldwide under the Berne Convention. May not be copied or distributed without prior written permission by the publisher. If you have this book or an electronic document and didn't pay for it, then the author didn't get a fair share. Please consider paying for your copy. Thank you!

Printed in the United States of America

ISBN 978-1475192056

Contents

Foreward

By Deanna R. Miller, RN MSN/Ed HCE

Confusion, forgetfulness, short-term memory loss, call it what you will, but each of us has been around someone that may be experiencing signs and symptoms of dementia. During my 23 years as a clinician, I have seen patients that were diagnosed with Alzheimer's disease and dementia because they just could not reason or had difficulty with their short-term memory. For many years I accepted those two diagnoses without question. Today, I know that these patients were given a very broad diagnosis for their symptoms, that in reality, probably was dementia with Lewy bodies or DLB.

So, we ask ourselves, "Does it really matter what kind of dementia an individual has?" The short answer to this question is, "absolutely." By determining the type of dementia that an individual suffers with early on in the disease process will not only pave a more positive path for treatment but will also help with research in finding a cure for these various types of diseases. True diagnosis of the condition can make for the best chances for a better quality of life.

In "Lewy Body Dementia: Causes, Tests and Treatment Options," the authors provide the reader with an abundance of information that is easy to understand and can be applied to the lives of those that are affected by this disease whether they are friends or family. Anyone of any age can be affected by dementia. This disease process is not selective and it does not only happen to "old people." It is very important that if the symptoms begin in a friend or loved one that the necessary diagnostics be performed to assure that the person is not suffering from a temporary type of confusion or forgetfulness associated with medications or some other type of disease process. Although there is not a specific test that determines DLB, there is a battery of diagnostics that should be performed to eliminate other disease processes. These include laboratory work, mental assessment, neurological exams, and an electroencephalogram. It is a diagnosis of elimination in that all other possible diseases are ruled out.

"Lewy Body Dementia: Causes, Tests, and Treatment Options" is one of the best books on the market today. As a valuable tool for the nurse, nursing assistant, patient, family member and physician, "Lewy Body Dementia: Causes, Tests, and Treatment Options" will provide all with the information that is needed to understand, treat and provide compassionate care to the individual that suffers from this devastating disease.

In the early stages of any type of dementia, no one is more frustrated than the individual that is afflicted. As the disease progresses you must always keep in mind that the individual affected has a story…they have a history. They were once someone's baby that was held in the arms of a caring mother. They were once the spouse of a loving companion. They were once the mother that cared for and nurtured her children. They are a human being with feelings and needs that must be met. Take care of our friends and family members that suffer from DLB or other types of mentally debilitating illnesses.

Introduction

It has been estimated that 1.3 million people in the United States have Lewy Body Dementia, also known as dementia with Lewy bodies or DLB. Its symptoms mimic other, better known, cognitive function illnesses like Alzheimer's. It is an umbrella term that is used to describe either of two diagnosis; Dementia with Lewy bodies and Parkinson's disease dementia. Lewy bodies, for which the condition is named, are abnormal round chemicals in the brain, particularly in the regions that control movement and thinking. Where these Lewy bodies are found is the reason that it affects cognitive function and the ability to move well, and what links it to being similar to Alzheimer's and Parkinson's.

While the cause is yet to be known, LBD is tied to both Alzheimer's and Parkinson's disease. Lewy bodies can have one of the same proteins that are associated with Parkinson's disease and are often in the brains of those who have rare dementias. Those with Lewy bodies that are found in the brain can also have the same tangles and plaques that are associated with Alzheimer's disease.

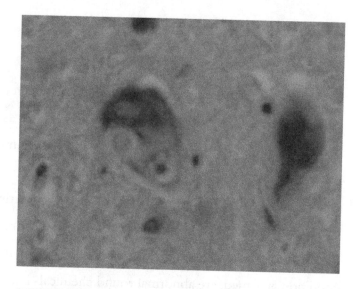

Lewy bodies are the pathophysiological characteristic of the disease

With these similarities, LBD is often put in the same categories and are thought to be related. Dementia with Lewy bodies and Alzheimer's disease can both be diagnosed in the same individual in some cases. People who are male, older than 60 years of age, and have a family history of Lewy Body

Dementia are more prone to have an increased risk factor for the disease, according to the Mayo Clinic.

Some medications that are taken for other illnesses may interact unfavorably with the symptoms of DLB. Diphenhydramine, dimenhydrinate, surgical anesthetics, anticholinergics, benzodiazepines, and older antidepressants may heighten the sedation, confusion, or motor impairment of Lewy Body Dementia. Dopamine agonists, anticholinergics, and amantadine may relieve Parkinson's disease symptoms but increase the hallucinations, delusions, and confusion of DLB. If you are going to have surgery or are taking any long-term medication for a chronic condition, tell your healthcare provider. Alternative medication may be provided.

There can be physical and mental symptoms with DLB. Symptoms will vary depending on the person and their immediate health. Not all DLB patients will exhibit all signs, nor will they have the same progression rate. Talk to support care about living with the condition or caring for someone with the condition to get a more accurate view on your individual case.

Physical symptoms of the condition include slowed movements, tremors of the extremities, shuffling gait, and rigid muscle tension. These signs are similar to those found in Parkinson's disease. There can be sleep issues and disturbances that may cause you or your loved one to act out dreams while still asleep. There are several vision symptoms for dementia with Lewy bodies including hallucinating shapes, people, animals, or colors that are not there. These hallucinations may be one of the earliest symptoms of the condition that you may be able to notice.

Psychological signs can be troubling and may include delusions, attention-span problems, and other cognitive problems. Delusions may make the person feel false thoughts against another person or about a particular situation or event. There can be confusion, short attention span, and the loss of some memories— like with Alzheimer's. Attention may be lowered and coincide with staring off into space, drowsiness, lethargy, and speech that is not organized properly. Rapid eye movement (REM) sleep is often quite disturbed, with loved ones unable to get a good night's sleep.

Getting a Diagnosis

With the vague tendencies of early dementia, it is sometimes difficult to get the correct diagnosis. It may be years before the proper type of dementia is spotted in a loved one. While some dementia is reversible, others are not, so finding the correct dementia type as soon as possible can be beneficial to you. Any change in cognitive function, memory, or thinking should be reported to a healthcare professional at your earliest convenience. There can be illnesses and medications that bring on dementia-like symptoms. Even certain vitamin deficiencies can mimic the condition. All of these are easily treated and you may be able to go on living without dementia symptoms. However, if this is not the case, then for non-curable dementia at least the accurate diagnosis can lead to the best appropriate treatment. Most non-curable dementia is seen in those who are over 50, but some have been seen in those who are in their 40s.

Treatment Options

Since there is no definite cure for the condition, Lewy Body Dementia is treated with a variety of options. You and your loved ones have the choice of medications, non-drug therapies, and alternative medicine options. Thinking about each of these treatment choices thoroughly can help you make a truly informed decision to your long-term health. Keep in mind, you'll need to have a definite diagnosis of the condition to know which medication and therapy options will be right for your situation.

Medications

There are several medications that are used for dementia with Lewy bodies. These are medications that are typically used to treat Alzheimer's and Parkinson's. Alzheimer's medications like cholinesterase inhibitors increase the amount of neurotransmitters in the brain. These are what researchers believe are responsible for good memory and judgment. Drugs in this class improve alertness. They may lower the degree and frequency of hallucinations as well. Cholinesterase inhibitors may increase salivation and tearing, increase urination frequency, and result in gastrointestinal upset. Antipsychotics tend to be used – with caution – to reduce hallucinations and delusions in Lewy Body Dementia. There are some serious issues with using drugs in this class for loved ones with the condition, and if they are considered as a treatment option, they should be carefully considered. Medications that are used to treat Parkinson's disease have the ability to lower the amount of muscular and movement symptoms in Dementia with Lewy bodies. Side effects of this type of medication can include an increase in delusions, hallucinations, and range of confusion.

Non-Drug Therapies

Non-drug therapies may appeal more to those who are hoping to forego medication. There are many lifestyle changes that can be done to help increase function, focus, and relaxation. You or your loved one may simplify tasks into smaller parts, reduce the clutter in your life, and reduce the levels of noise. Those three items can help focus and give a sound structure to the routine. By not correcting your loved one or badgering them with questions, you are helping to create a harmonious environment without unsettling them and causing them increased anxiety.

Alternative Medicine Options

Anytime you can increase restful relaxation and put your body into a better, calmer state, your body can lessen its symptoms. Frustration can heighten the affect that symptoms have on you or a loved one. Therefore, any type of relaxation therapy such as massage, aromatherapy, acupressure, and acupuncture, may help in increasing the quality of life. Breathing exercises may also help.

Caregiver Tips

Caring for a loved one with Lewy Body Dementia can be tricky since everyone will have slightly varying symptoms and will have their condition progress differently. There are some good tricks to help have a more harmonious lifestyle with the condition. Since anxiety, confusion, and behavior all seem to worsen during the nighttime hours, create a routine for the evening, lowering the level of noise and activity. Setting up a strict routine without too much variance can increase a sense of safety and lower anxiety. Another anxiety-lowering lifestyle change is to reduce caffeine during the day. Exercise may help both mood and symptoms. Exercise can also have beneficial effects on depression symptoms, motor skills, cardiovascular health, and strength. Try to use touch conversation, where you touch your loved one's arm or shoulder while speaking to them. Touch can work as a calming agent. Speaking slowly, articulately, and simply can help their understanding. Always wait for them to reply without rushing them. Gesturing with your hands can help increase their understanding of what you are saying.

Prognosis

According to the Lewy Body Dementia Association, the long-term prognosis for the condition will vary from person to person. Each prognosis is different due to the person's general health or if there are other underlying conditions coexisting with the Lewy body dementia. The condition will progress differently from person to person as well. There is not a way to properly determine the length of life after a diagnosis or how quickly the onset of symptom progression will be. However, there are averages that can help give a ballpark estimate. For the majority of loved ones with the condition, the duration of the illness is five to eight years after the symptoms begin. Some individuals may fall anywhere between two years and twenty years after symptoms begin.

Do You Tell Loved Ones They Have Lewy Body Dementia?

One of the most asked questions concerning this condition is whether or not to tell the person they have Lewy Body Dementia. Disclosure will ultimately be left up to the caregiver, but some things that may influence the decision include temperament and cognitive ability. There have been studies where there have been indications that people can find relief in knowing that their symptoms are real and their condition has a name. True diagnosis of the condition can make for the best chances for a better quality of life and the best treatment plan.

There is research being done to find out more about this condition. The National Institute of Neurological Disorders and Stroke (NINDS) does much of this research. It is done typically through grants given to medical institutes and facilities. Scientists are looking into the genetic roots of dementia with Lewy bodies including alpha-synuclein accumulation and the direct cause of how the Lewy bodies can give off symptoms of the condition. Researchers are hoping to find better treatment options, ways to prevent the progression of symptoms, and ultimately find a cure for it.

Diagnosis of Lewy Body Dementia

Lewy Body Dementia accounts for around 10 to 15 percent of diagnosed dementias. This low prevalence and the similarity of the disease to Alzheimer's and Parkinson's present issues with confirming a diagnosis of the disease. Up until the 1990s, actual confirmation of the diagnosis was only available in post-mortem autopsy. Up to 80 percent of people suffering from Lewy Body Dementia receive a diagnosis for a different form of dementia before their actual diagnosis is found. The overlapping symptoms with Parkinson's and Alzheimer's, which are much more prevalent, play a large role in the misdiagnosis of DLB. With numbers of DLB diagnoses growing to over 1 million in the United States alone, it has become one of the most prevalent forms of dementia, and education on symptoms and helping your doctor properly diagnosing the disease are extremely important.

Differences between Lewy Body Dementia and Alzheimer's

Alzheimer's disease is a single disease in which some people may or may not have dementia as a symptom. Alzheimer's disease causes tangles and plaques on the brain in abnormal quantities, interfering with brain function. It has been known to increase the timeframe of brain aging. Alzheimer's is the most known and widespread form of dementia, with Lewy Body Dementia being second. About seventy percent of all individuals with dementia will have Alzheimer's. The main differences between Dementia with Lewy bodies and Alzheimer's is where the cognitive function decline lies. In Alzheimer's disease the decline is in memory most prominently. In Dementia with Lewy bodies, the decline is in thinking, problem solving, and the ability to reason. Hallucinations are symptoms of DLB in the beginning stages, while it is not a symptom of Alzheimer's until much later in the progression of that condition. REM sleep can be fine in an Alzheimer's patient, while a Lewy Body Disease patient is most likely going to have sleep disturbances. These are the main polarities to the two conditions.

Differences between Lewy Body Dementia and Parkinson's Disease Dementia

Those with Parkinson's disease have a chance to develop what is known as Parkinson's Disease Dementia, or PDD. Those over 65 years of age have a greater risk, with ten percent of those between 50 and 60 years of age already developing PDD. PDD and Dementia with Lewy bodies differ in the symptoms that present themselves first. If the motor skill decline is present before the cognitive decline, experts call it PDD. If the cognitive decline is showing up prior to the motor symptoms, typically it is referred to as Lewy Body Dementia. Symptoms of PDD include mental inflexibility, mental clarity degeneration, visuospatial function worsening, hallucinations, memory impairment, blank stares, and daytime sleepiness. PDD is progressive, lasting several years after the symptoms begin. Cholinesterase inhibitors can be used to treat the condition with some success.

Other Forms of Dementia

A couple of other forms of dementia should be noted. Knowing the symptoms and aspects of these can help you and your doctor more easily distinguish them from PDD, Alzheimer's, and DLB. These are frontotemporal dementia, dementia from Huntington's, infectious disease induced dementia, and vascular dementia.

Frontotemporal Dementia

Frontotemporal dementia, or FTD, is a condition that includes many disorders. With FTD, the symptoms are compulsive behavior, apathy, personality changes, lack of awareness of their condition, and a personal hygiene decline. Their behavior may be inappropriate. FTD may include changes with the person's speech, language, and movement. FTD is diagnosed from a medical exam and a brain imaging or scanning. There may be signs of deterioration of the temporal or the frontal lobes. While there is no definite cure for the condition, there are treatments and therapies that can be done to help increase the quality of life.

Infectious Disease Induced Dementia

Viruses and bacteria can get into the brain and cause a few forms of dementia. One of these, Creutzfeldt-Jakob disease, is a rare infectious disease induced dementia type. Dementia from an infectious disease is spread through a protein called a prion. These invade the brain, destroying nerve cells, making the progression of memory problems and other cognitive issues quicker than with traditional, more mainstream, conditions like Alzheimer's and Dementia with Lewy bodies. While the rare condition can be diagnosed through medical history and symptoms, only an autopsy will definitively confirm it. Upon autopsy, the brain tissue will be found to have holes from the destruction of the cells.

Dementia from Huntington's Disease

Dementia may also come from the progression of Huntington's disease, which is a fatal condition of brain nerve cells. It is genetic, and typically isn't showing signs until middle age. There are only 30,000 Huntington's cases in the United States. Signs are similar to Alzheimer's in that there is memory loss, mood swings, disorientation, and personality changes. Also, like Parkinson's dementia, there are irregular and jerky movements, and the loss of the abilities to talk and walk. Huntington's disease has no definite cure or real treatment options currently, and the long-term prognosis is to increase the quality of life while alive. It can be determined by a simple blood test, looking for the defective gene.

Vascular Dementia

When there are a series of small strokes in the brain that affect function, it is called vascular dementia. The strokes deprive the brain of oxygen and nutrients, leaving behind symptoms of dementia. These signs include a shuffling gait, disorientation with familiar settings, incontinence, the inability to follow instructions, and inappropriate laughing or crying. There may be inability to handle money. Some of the risk factors for vascular dementia include smoking cigarettes, high cholesterol (hypercholesterolemia), and high blood pressure (hypertension). Vascular dementia can be seen easily on a MRI or CT scan if it's from a cerebrovascular cause. Having a history of any of the risk factors can help lead to its diagnosis. Treating some of these risk factors can help slow the dementia's progression. There are no approved medications for vascular dementia, although Aricept, the popular Alzheimer's drug, is often used. In a 2006 study of a clinical trial group, there were 11 deaths of vascular dementia patients taking Aricept, as opposed to none in the control group that was not taking the drug.

Difficulties in Diagnosing DLB for Doctors and Families

The most limiting factor in the diagnosis of DLB is the lack of one specific test that can confirm the disease. The second major issue is the nature of the disease which puts observed symptoms as a mixture of Alzheimer's and Parkinson's. The lack of knowledge of the disease outside of specialty doctors also plays a role. Most people only visit a primary care physician, except in the case of an emergency or extremely unusual event. The difficulty this presents is in the specialized nature of diagnosing DLB. General practitioner doctors need an enormous amount of medical information on hand to deal with the broad spectrum of human illness, and unfortunately this can be an issue when trying to diagnose a more obscure disease.

More specifically, DLB causes the person to have symptoms similar to Parkinson's in that they may suffer slower and stiffer movement, but unlike Parkinson's they will not suffer from tremors. This can be overlooked by doctors who are unaware of DLB and attributed to simply a result of aging. The Lewy Body Dementia Association conducted surveys concerning the diagnostic process that DLB sufferers and caregivers went through, and found that over half of DLB patients went through over 10 doctor visits before reaching a diagnosis, and almost a third did not receive the diagnosis within a year of first reporting symptoms. You can unfortunately expect a long and difficult journey when going through the diagnostic process unless you choose your physician with care and arm yourself with information about the disease. Later sections in this book offer advice on choosing physicians and offer tips for your appointments.

Diagnostic Criteria for DLB

There is not a single, definitive test for DLB. Diagnosing the disease requires testing to narrow down the possible causes and elimination of other possible causes until DLB is the definitive diagnosis. Like most diseases, the diagnostic process starts with reporting of the symptoms by the one suffering from the disease, or friends and family.

There are not many factors that predispose someone to developing DLB. The disease is still relatively new, and research into it is still ongoing. Like Alzheimer's, the disease is more likely in older people. It is also showing possibilities of a genetic connection and more likely to occur in males, but neither is conclusive as of yet. The disease also tends to show in people with other dementia disorders, such as those described above. The symptoms of DLB will always include dementia, a progressive decline in mental function. In addition to dementia, the doctor will usually need to see symptoms of: recurring and detailed visual hallucinations; symptoms akin to Parkinson's disease; and changes in level of cognitive function. One or two of the secondary symptoms is usually enough to at least indicate possible or probable DLB.

Other symptoms can also suggest DLB. When a symptom is described as suggestive, it means it is frequent enough in a disease to indicate a possibility of it, but is not enough on its own if most of the core symptoms do not exist to point towards a high probability. Suggestive symptoms for DLB include REM sleep disorder, active dreams and severe neuroleptic sensitivity. REM disorder can present with twitching and movement during sleep, and neuroleptic sensitivity causes people with DLB to suffer severe reactions to neuroleptic medicine. If you or your family member has had an allergic reaction to any medication, be sure to tell your doctor.

Active Dreams (RBD) and Lewy Body Dementia

Active dreams refer to the symptom of the Rapid Eye Movement sleep behavior disorder (RBD) whereby the patient acts out what happens in a dream. Normally, when a person is in the REM state, the eyes tend to move frantically, causing the eyelids to flutter while the rest of the body is in a restrained state. Due to this, a person will relax even if the dream is already in an active sequence. For RBD sufferers, the movement restriction is not in force. A person goes into a state called active dreaming, where a patient acts out exactly as he does in the dream and there are moments when things become violent.

Active dreaming is one of the preliminary symptoms of Lewy Body Dementia or LBD. About 50% of people who are having active dreams develop LBD in later life. This sleeping disorder continues to pester patients as the dementia worsens and at advanced states, hallucinations and delusions accompany these active dreams. As the defining symptom that is very common with LBD, a patient can suffer from RBD years before the cognitive dysfunction shows.

This sleeping disorder is difficult to deal with as it can disrupt the sleep of the patient. In RBD, the patient feels as if a dream is realistic although everything due to the relative vividness of the dream. There is also an observable decline in the patient's ability to control all of his body functions.

Having active dreams is a very common symptom in LBD, so people who are already experiencing this sleeping disorder have an early warning that they are susceptible to LBD. The best way to prevent the onset of dementia early on is to avoid moments of extreme stress. For those who are planning to undergo an elective surgery or those who take drugs that are not recommended for LBD patients, it would be better to avoid these things altogether. Sharing the patient's RBD symptoms with your doctor is also worth mentioning, as it may save a loved one from developing early dementia.

When a person experiences active dreaming, that individual wouldn't know or remember what happened. Since the person is still in a subconscious state and, due to RBD, his movement is not restricted, it would be possible to for the patient to hurt himself and his bed partner.

Peter, whose wife Annique suffers from LBD, recalls the times when he experienced active dreams of his wife when she tried to hit him while asleep. The morning after, Annique did not remember anything about the incident.

Due to the active dreamer's mobility, it is vital to make sure that the patient is sleeping in a safe environment. Placing the bed in a corner (with the active dreamer sleeping close to the wall) which is far from the window is important, as well as removing objects that can cause injury away from the bedside table. It would also be advisable to add some padding to the headboard and wall.

A number of symptoms and signs are also either supportive or occur in people with DLB. Having these symptoms and signs is not enough to even suggest a possibility of DLB on their own, but they help to support a diagnosis of the disease if the possibility already exists. These include depression, delusions, frequent falling, losses of consciousness, and severe autonomic dysfunction.

After the reporting of the symptoms, there will still be several possible causes. A number of different tests are a possibility once there are signs of impaired brain function. Tests range from simple procedures like reflex tests to tests involving modern medical equipment such as MRIs. The doctor may perform a neurological exam designed to test the reflexes, eye movements, sense of balance, and sense of touch of the patient. This test is used for conditions like Parkinson's, cancer, and strokes in addition to being relevant for DLB. It will help determine if the disease is also affecting physical function as well as mental function, which helps the diagnostic process.

You or your loved one will likely receive a mental assessment exam. These tests can take anywhere from 10 minutes to several hours depending on the detail of the exam. The assessment will help determine if brain function is suffering from any decline compared to where it should be for the person's age and education level. The specific types of decline can help indicate the disease as well.

You will likely have some blood tests and other forms of lab work done. These are done to rule out other possibilities for mental decline, such as a vitamin B-12 deficiency and thyroid malfunction. Other tests will include EEGs and brain scans. The EEG is an analysis of the electrical activity in the brain, which is used to rule out diseases involving seizures; specific abnormalities in the Q-T section of the test have been linked to DLB. The brain scan looks for issues such as tumors and strokes that could explain a change in brain activity.

These tests should all combine to eliminate other possibilities if DLB is the source of the person's suffering. Research is ongoing to find more conclusive tests that can help diagnose DLB with less testing and earlier after symptoms are reported.

Testing for Lewy Body Dementia

Testing for the condition consists of checking you or your loved one for a decline in thinking ability. If you have a cognitive decline as well as either Parkinson's-like signs, visual hallucinations, or wavering alertness, doctors will start the elimination process to rule out everything else but the condition. There is not a solitary test for the disease, so other diseases must be ruled out. It is a diagnosis of exclusion. There are several tests that may be helpful in leading to a diagnosis, however. These include laboratory work, mental assessment, neurological exams, and an electroencephalogram (EEG).

Laboratory Work

Some brain function problems can be linked to vitamin deficiencies or thyroid issues. Your doctor will do simple lab tests that include blood work to check for these types of problems. Typically, all this will involve is a needle inserted into a vein; and a few vials of blood taken. While it can be uncomfortable and you may experience bleeding afterwards or bruising, it is a relatively painless procedure. If the symptoms are linked to vitamin deficiencies or a thyroid that is not functioning properly, they can treat that as well. Vitamin B-12 deficiencies, which can cause some brain function problems. Thyroid problems are easily treated with the patient resuming most of their normal activities afterward.

Mental Ability Assessment

Most mental ability testing will take between 10 minutes to several hours of your time. Checking for memory loss can be fast, while checking for neuropsychiatric abnormalities can take much longer. These results are compared to results from others in your age bracket and your education background. This comparison can help the doctors assess if your mental status is declining. It is helpful to go in as soon as possible for a mental assessment, so that a baseline can be taken. These baselines are helpful if there is additional decline through the years.

Neurological Exams

One of the most important of the physical tests done for the diagnosis includes checking for other conditions or items that may affect the function of the brain. Doctors look for balance, eye movements, reflexes, and your sense of touch. They may do brain scans such as a CT or an MRI to see if there is any bleeding or if there has been a stroke. They may also able to tell if there is a tumor in the brain from these imaging tests.

Electroencephalogram

The electroencephalogram, or EEG, can be a vital part of the diagnostic process, especially if confusion is not constant, i.e. it comes and goes. An EEG can check to see if the symptoms you or your loved one are experiencing are due to Lewy Body Dementia or if they are something more rare, like Creutzfeldt-Jakob disease. While the EEG can make the doctor suspect Creutzfeldt-Jakob disease, again, the definitive signs can only be seen after death. The test is painless and only records the brain's electrical activity by small electrodes that are attached temporarily for the test.

The DLB Healthcare Appointment

When it comes to your **primary care physician,** choosing one who has experience in dealing with LBD and has working knowledge of the disease is important. There is no comprehensive list of doctors with knowledge of LBD, and there is no certification for dealing with the disease. Asking on LBD support forums for information on local doctors with a history of treating LBD can often provide good leads. Resources such as the Lewy Body Dementia Association, the Alzheimer's Association, and the Mayo Clinic include support for LBD and can offer information on how to choose a primary doctor.

Dealing with the progression of the Parkinsonism involved in LBD presents negative changes to the quality of life experienced by the sufferer and those around them. **Occupational therapists** can help alleviate this stress by giving instructions on how to handle activities of daily life while suffering from limitations. Their services are given to a wide range of people with disabilities, including those with neurological symptoms such as LBD or Parkinson's. Occupational therapists are particularly helpful in maintaining independence, which can help improve quality of life and levels of happiness in a person.

Physical therapists come in a large number of varieties, but two specialties in particular are beneficial for LBD patients: PTs with training for neurological diseases, and those experienced with elderly patients. Therapists with specialization in neurological diseases regularly treat patients who have impairments in brain function, and help them to regain mobility and strength, as well as often improving mental function through exercise. Since patients suffering from LBD, Alzheimer's, and Parkinson's are often elderly, physical therapists with a focus in treating the elderly deal with the diseases on a regular basis. Both are valid options when seeking a physical therapist, and a therapist who holds specialties in both fields will be particularly useful.

In addition to a primary care doctor who is knowledgeable of LBD, you will likely want to find a good **neurologist.** These doctors specialize in the research and treatment of conditions that impact cognitive function. Neurologists have to go through a specialized board to receive their certification in the field, ensuring they are up to date on the latest treatments and techniques. A neurologist is not a replacement for a primary care doctor, who helps manage your overall health, but their expertise in the field as part of a comprehensive treatment program can be invaluable.

With the wide range of symptoms in each LBD case, it is important to follow an overall guideline of addressing every symptom in some form. If the LBD patient is having difficulties giving or receiving communication, then a **speech therapist** could be able to help. If the patient is dealing with the REM sleep disorder common in LDB, a **sleep specialist** should be sought. **Psychiatrists** can also help with the cognitive problems and disorientation issues presented in dementia. The rule of thumb should be that if a symptom exists, and it is remotely connected to LBD, bring it up with your primary care doctor and ask if there are specialists they can recommend to manage the issue.

Preparing yourself or a loved one for that appointment is easier when you know in advance what to expect. Your family or general care doctor may lead you to a psychiatrist or a neurologist. There are things that you can do to make the best possible outcome from the appointment and things that you should be expecting of the doctor. The appointment can be made for just the suspected dementia patient or as a group with friends and family members. Typically, the more people that are there, the easier it is to get a well-rounded view of the patient and their true symptoms and signs.

Make a list early on that includes everything you want to cover with the doctor. Also make a some lists of all the important items the doctor will need while you or a loved one is in with the doctor at the appointment. These lists should contain items such as questions, your medications, and symptoms. Make one list of detailed symptoms. Make another that includes every drug you are taking or have taken, including dosages. These drugs should also include nonprescription ones, like over-the-counter medication, supplements, vitamins, and herbals. The list of questions should include things like inquiring about the testing, the treatment options, prognosis, etc.

Things to Expect From Your Doctor at Your DLB Appointment

Your doctor will question you and anyone who is with you about your condition. They will want to review your list of medications. Whether you have them or not, your doctor will ask you about hallucinations. They will take a detailed history on any head trauma, brain problems, or other aspect that could be a key factor in your diagnosis. These keys can include depression, stroke, or alcohol abuse. Lastly, they are going to make sure they fully understand your personality, behavior, and memory. Asking those who are there with you can help bring out subtle changes that you may have missed.

Treatment Options for Lewy Body Dementia

Treatment for Dementia with Lewy Bodies is a complex and multi-faceted process. There is no definite cure for the disease. The options for DLB treatment fall into two categories: medical treatments to mitigate symptoms of the disease, and therapy and care options to ease suffering and improve function as the disease progresses. While DLB will have a dramatic impact on the lives of those suffering and their families, there is still hope for many happy and active years together with proper care.

Medical Treatments for DLB

There are a number of medical treatments that can help alleviate a variety of the symptoms of DLB. No drugs as of yet have been shown to have an effect on slowing down the progression of DLB, but reduction of cognitive impairment, hallucinations, sleeping issues, and Parkinsonism is possible.

Treatment for the hallucinations and delusions associated with DLB with pharmaceuticals is an especially tricky process due to the prevalence of severe neuroleptic sensitivity in DLB sufferers. Neuroleptic sensitivity causes the more common drugs for hallucinations, usually used to treat Alzheimer's disease, to exacerbate the problems associated with DLB and can cause other severe side-effects. These changes can become irreversible if treatment with neuroleptics is continued for too long. Before more knowledge was gained on LBD, the common misdiagnoses of the disease as Alzheimer's led to many people being given neuroleptics. Now there are several options in lieu of them for DLB sufferers.

Cholinesterase Inhibitors

Cholinesterase inhibitors are used to treat some of the cognitive symptoms and behavioral impairment in diseases such as Alzheimer's and LBD. There are several drugs that qualify as cholinesterase inhibitors, listed with the brand name first, followed by the generic name in parenthesis: Aricept and Aricept ODT (Donepezil), Cognex (tacrine), Razadyne and Razadyne ER (galantamine), and Exelon (rivastigmine). The inhibitors combine with cholinesterase in the brain in order to block it, which causes higher level of the neurotransmitter acetylcholine (ACh) in the synapses. Cholinesterase is produced in cholinergic synapses, and is responsible for acetylcholine breakdown. Stopping the cholinesterase from acting on the acetylcholine results in improving cognitive function.

Cholinesterase inhibitors occur naturally as venoms and poisons that act as nerve agents. The compounds act on the autonomic nervous system and can cause low blood pressure (hypotension), arrhythmia, SLUDGE syndrome (salivation, lacrimation, urination, defecation, gastrointestinal upset and Emesis), long-lasting muscle contraction, constriction of air passages in the respiratory tract, and increased activity in the GI tract. The poisonous nature requires a titration phase when the drug is administered to treat cognitive symptoms, which is a slow and steady increase of the dosage from a low starting point.

Side effects of Cholinesterase inhibitors include ALT (alanine transaminase) elevation in the liver, mild to moderate gastrointestinal upsets, fatigue, dizziness, somnolence, diarrhea, nausea, muscle cramping, and vomiting. Nausea, vomiting, and diarrhea constitute most of the reported side effects, but were seen to decrease once the titration phase of the drug was finished. The dizziness did pose an increased risk for falling, which is a concern for people suffering from the diseases the drug treats due to Parkinsonism.

Levodopa:

Levodopa, or L-DOPA (L-3,4-dihydroxyphenylalanine), is a drug used to treat abnormally low dopamine levels that occur in diseases like Parkinson's and LBD. Levodopa is produced normally in humans and other animals as a precursor to the neurotransmitters dopamine, norepinephrine, and epinephrine. Levodopa is separated from the neurotransmitters by its ability to cross the blood-brain barrier, which allows it to function as a medical treatment to increase dopamine levels in the brain. Vitamin B6 is part of the process the body uses to convert Levodopa into dopamine, so it may be given along with levodopa to facilitate the reaction.

The drug is still primarily used as a treatment for Parkinson's disease, but has shown some promise in helping DLB sufferers. The drug was shown to be about half as effective for DLB patients as it is for PD patients in improving scores on the UPDRS III (Unified Parkinson's Disease Rating Scale) test. Despite the small improvements gained by levodopa, it is one of the first drugs to show at least a significant amount of improvement in the capability of DLB sufferers to function. The drug also has a more pronounced effect when given in earlier stages of the disease.

Possible side effects of L-dopa include at least the following: Hypotension in high doses, rare occurrences of arrhythmia, nausea that can be reduced by taking the drug with food, hair loss, gastrointestinal bleeding, insomnia, auditory and visual hallucinations, narcolepsy, somnolence, hair loss, disorientation, and confusion. Prolonged usage of levodopa can result in dysregulation of dopamine production (dopamine dysregulation syndrome), serotonin depletion, Dyskinesia, and reductions in the effectiveness of the drug. The list of side effects is long, but is relatively low compared to other treatments used for Parkinson's and DLB.

Antipsychotics

Antipsychotic medication is used regularly to treat hallucinations and delusions in people who suffer from certain mental diseases, such as schizophrenia, and can help reduce these symptoms in Alzheimer's patients. Typical antipsychotics, also known as neuroleptics, include chlorpromazine, droperidol, haloperidol, loxapine, and several more. These typical antipsychotics should not be prescribed to someone suffering from DLB due to around 50 percent of them having neuroleptic sensitivity. This causes increased cognitive impairment, sedation, increased Parkinsonism, and in rare cases it may cause the development of Neuroleptic Malignant Syndrome (NMS). NMS manifests as fever, stiffness in the muscles, kidney failure, and death.

If you or your loved one are diagnosed with a different dementia-related condition and suffer adverse effects from a typical neuroleptic, notifying your doctor may help lead to a proper diagnosis of DLB. Many people currently diagnosed with DLB have suffered from issues with neuroleptics prior to the correct diagnosis, making this a serious problem to be concerned with and watchful of for the health of yourself or your loved ones.

There are atypical antipsychotic medications doctors can prescribe in order to mitigate the hallucinations involved in DLB. The list includes aripiprazole, clozapine, fluoxetine, risperidone, and quetiapine. Many have strong side effects and need careful monitoring of the dosage and the patient. Clozapine requires frequent blood tests to check for potential problems, and quetiapine and clozapine (brand name Seroquel and Abilify respectively) need to be administered at low doses and for short periods of time to avoid possible side effects.

Clozapine and quetiapine are the most commonly prescribed antipsychotics to DLB sufferers. Clozapine has been shown to cause issues due to anticholinergic affects and the risk for agranulocytosis, a condition that suppresses the immune system by lowering specific type of white blood cell count. As such, quetiapine is becoming the more likely medicine of choice when antipsychotics are deemed necessary. The drugs risperidone and olanzapine have serious side effects associated with them, such as increased Parkinsonism, high levels of sedation, and orthostatic hypotension. As such, they should be avoided without good reason provided by a medical professional.

Antipsychotic Medication Warning

As many as half of the people that are given antipsychotic medications for the condition have the risk to experience many severe side effects. These serious side effects include profound sedation, severe neuroleptic sensitivity, cognitive function worsening, symptoms that mimic neuroleptic malignant syndrome (NMS), and heightened or irreversible Parkinsonism.

All antipsychotics have been shown to have adverse effects in elderly patients with dementia, including increased risk of death. The usage of antipsychotics should therefore involve a serious discussion with the doctor, patient, and loved ones in order to assess if the possible reduction in behavioral symptoms is worth the associated side effects and other risks of the medication. If it is decided that antipsychotics are the best course of action, the doctor should be kept aware of any changes or the occurrence of known side effects immediately.

Melatonin and Clonazepam

DLB sufferers often have symptoms of REM sleep disorder. This occurs in the stages of sleep where dreaming is most vivid, and in DLB the disorder can result in twitching and full movement of the person while asleep. This can be hazardous to the safety of the sufferer and those around them, so medicinal treatment is given to reduce the symptoms, typically in the form of melatonin and clonazepam.

Melatonin is a naturally occurring chemical that helps regulate sleep patterns. The hormone is produced in the pineal gland, and causes drowsiness and lower body temperature. Melatonin production naturally decreases with age, making it especially effective as a treatment for DLB patients who are typically older. Melatonin also has been shown to increase learning capabilities in mice, and as such has been given to Alzheimer's patients to help them retain information. The chemical prevents hyper phosphorylation of the tau protein in mice, which causes the neurofibrillary tangles that are common in Alzheimer's and DLB.

As Melatonin occurs naturally in humans, its side effects are not very extreme. Short term side effects include grogginess and drowsiness, nausea, intense dreaming, irritability, and hypothermia. As it is intended to help facilitate sleep, care should be taken when operating heavy machinery while taking melatonin. Long-term usage has not been shown to cause serious side effects, though conclusive studies have not been performed. There are extended release versions of the pills available. Melatonin is readily bought over the counter in the United States, but be sure to inform your doctor if you decide to start on any regular medication, as drug interactions may be potentially harmful.

Warning

Sleep disorders—especially if the patient is experiencing active dreams (thrashing, or yelling in their sleep)—is one of the early warning signs of dementia. Stressful events, such as surgery, can make dementia worse. Therefore, you should consult with an expert on LBD before undertaking any surgery—especially if you are experiencing active dreams.

Clonazepam, often given under the brand name Klonopin, is a benzodiazepine drug that has effect as a muscle relaxer and as a hypnotic. Normal doses of clonazepam are used mainly to treat epilepsy, but the drug is also used for nervous and sleep disorders such as restless leg syndrome and REM sleep disorder when administered at low doses. Clonazepam is also used to treat feelings of restlessness and inability to sit still, commonly associated with antipsychotic medication.

As opposed to melatonin, Clonazepam has a long list of side effects. In order of frequency, the common side effects are: drowsiness, impaired cognitive and motor function, euphoria, irritability, feelings of restlessness and compulsion to move, loss of motivation, decreased sexual drive, dizziness, loss of coordination and balance, hallucinations, loss of short-term memory, hangover-like symptoms, and rebound insomnia when discontinuing the drug suddenly. Rare but serious side effects include changes in personality, confusion, ataxia, psychiatric and psychological changes, severe dysphoria, a decrease in blood platelets (thrombocytopenia) leading to bleeding issues, psychosis, incontinence, and manic behaviorisms such as rage and impulsivity.

Long-term usage of clonazepam results in both tolerance and physical addiction. Discontinuing the drug suddenly results in withdrawal symptoms characteristic of benzodiazepine withdrawal such as psychosis, irritability, anxiety, and aggressiveness. This dependence can occur after a relatively short treatment time of just 2-4 weeks. Elderly patients are particularly susceptible to the dependency on clonazepam, as they metabolize the drug less quickly than younger people, and the elderly are more sensitive to the effects of benzodiazepines in general. The sedative effects can combine with the other common DLB medications, resulting in severe somnolence and lack of energy. Clonazepam has also seen frequent use as a recreational drug.

Drug Trials and Experimental Medicine

Dementia with Lewy bodies is a relatively new disease, and as such research is still currently ongoing in the pharmaceutical field to find new treatments that help alleviate or even cure the disease. As the name indicates, experimental medicines are generally less tested and can be potentially dangerous. For those who are not seeing results from other medications, it can be a possibility to look in to. Ask your doctor about available drug trials, and do not seek to join a drug trial independently without at least consulting your primary doctor.

Non-Medical Treatments

In addition to the drug treatments available, there are a number of therapy options available that help alleviate symptoms of DLB and ease suffering. Therapy options have a distinct advantage over medicinal treatments by not inducing side-effects common to most drugs. Options include physical therapy, speech therapy, occupational therapy, psychotherapy, and support groups for DLB. Therapy options do require more effort to bring about changes, and the apathy and disillusionment associated with

DLB can cause interest in them to wane and reduce their effectiveness.

Physical Therapy

Physical therapists work with patients suffering from a multitude of diseases, injuries, and disabilities. Their primary focus is on helping to improve motor function, such as walking and muscle strength. A physical therapist will usually have at least a Bachelor's degree in physical therapy, but most practicing PTs will have at least a Master's degree, and some hold doctorates. Your doctor will likely be able to point you to a well-trained and capable therapist.

Physical therapists have a number of specialties, including neurological specialists who work primarily with patients suffering from diseases such as cerebral palsy and Parkinson's disease. A neurologically specialized physical therapist can help the person perform better at activities of daily living, and studies have shown that regular exercise can slow the progression of dementia by promoting a good flow of blood and oxygen to the brain. Being better able to take care of themselves and being independently mobile can drastically improve quality of life for DLB sufferers.

Speech Therapy

The American Speech-Language-Hearing Association (ASHA) has undertaken recent studies in 2005 into the effectiveness of speech-related therapy on persons suffering from dementia, and found positive results. Speech therapy is not limited only to spoken communication, but also includes writing, reading, and gesturing. Dementia affects everyone in slightly different ways, but there is almost always an impairment of communication skills when dementia is involved. Problems communicating can be frustrating for both the sufferer and those around them. The ASHA states, "speech-language pathologists (SLPs) play a primary role in the screening, assessment, diagnosis, treatment, and research of dementia." The ASHA also says the role of speech therapists should be to help through all stages of dementia progression, and have an "ethical responsibility to do so."

Indicators of a possible need for speech therapy can be difficulty with appropriate word choices, significant delays in responses in conversation, trouble following directions, inappropriate behavior in social situations, and anger and frustration when attempting to communicate. Since DLB is a progressive disease that inhibits cognitive function, communication impediment is likely, and starting on a regimen of speech therapy earlier can help push back the onset of the communication issues. The therapists provide help to the family of the sufferer as well by giving instruction on more effective methods of communication.

Speech therapists also work with swallowing issues known as dysphagia that can cause difficulty eating or drinking. Dysphagia shows through sudden and inexplicable weight loss, difficulty swallowing, dehydration, and signs of malnutrition. Untreated, dysphagia can result in renal failure and further complications in the underlying disease.

Psychotherapy

Psychotherapy involves a number of options designed to promote or handle cognitive function and issues in patients suffering from dementia. The treatments focus on the psychological aspects of dealing with dementia, including cognitive, emotional, behavioral, and reality therapy. Psychological therapy is also an option for caregivers of dementia patients to help them cope with the difficulties associated with their role.

Reality therapy seeks to help ground the person suffering from dementia, which can cause disorientation and confusion. Methods include reminiscence therapy that uses physical objects that serve as memorabilia such as old photos and newspapers to elicit memories in the patient. The therapy also includes discussion with the patient about the current state of reality, intended to ground them in a concrete and stable world-view.

Dementia can be extremely emotionally upsetting, and providing an outlet and help dealing with these emotions is important to the well-being of the sufferer. Types of treatment include reminiscence therapy similar to the reality therapy above, sensory therapy that uses music and soothing sounds to induce relaxation, and normal psychological therapy to discuss the issues and concerns of the sufferer. Supportive psychotherapy is an emerging field of psychiatry that focuses on showing empathy and providing increased self-esteem. Emotion therapy has shown some effects on improving both the mood and cognition of patients, but the results are not conclusive. Inconclusive results do not indicate a lack of effectiveness, as measuring and analyzing data scientifically for mental and emotional issues is an inexact and complicated process.

Cognitive therapy also overlaps with reality therapy, but primarily focuses on improving cognitive ability by exercising the DLB patient's mental functions. This includes word exercises, visual activities, Stroop exercises, and other activities in methods such as Cognitive Retention Therapy. CRT itself is undergoing formal clinical trials currently, and might be an option if you seek it. Some negative side effects of cognitive therapy have been reported, such as increased frustration if the tasks seem too difficult to the patient.

Behavioral therapy deals with handling specific issues that arise due to dementia. Behavioral issues include more than just irritability and lashing out, comprising of almost anything that constitutes an action or difficulty controlling an action, such as incontinence or wandering due to confusion and psychomotor agitation. The approach is not overly successful in controlling behaviors beyond incontinence, but methods and information are continually improving.

Occupational Therapy

Occupational therapy specifically aims at health promotion and well-being through purposeful and meaningful activities, such as engagement in occupation. Occupational therapists work with people to maintain their ability to perform daily functions such as washing, cleaning, preparing food, and eating when inhibited by disease or disability. It can be seen as conjoined with physical therapy, as it does involve physically manipulating oneself and objects around them, but occupational therapy does include teaching on how to work around limitations. For example, switching phones in the house over to ones with oversized buttons can allow someone suffering from Parkinsonism, which causes twitching and loss of muscle control, to be better able to dial a phone number.

Occupational therapists also help improve the safety of an environment. The physical impairment a DLB sufferer goes through can cause a higher risk of falling, and as the majority of DLB sufferers are elderly this can present a risk of injury and death. By creating a safer environment, the OT can help a DLB patient become more independent, an important source of pride in many people.

The most important aspect of involving an occupational therapist in your treatment is the help they give in making someone as independent as possible. Extended care facilities are an option most families and sufferers want to avoid at all costs. The occupational therapist will work with the sufferer and caregivers to help establish routines and methods that minimize the care a DLB patient has to receive without pushing the patient too far. This freedom alleviates the burden from caregivers, and gives a sense of accomplishment.

Support Groups and Organizations

Having others who understand the situation you are going through there to support you and give you feedback is important, and support groups have been shown to be successful throughout a number of different conditions. DLB is no different, and many support groups and organizations exist that focus either primarily or extensively on DLB.

The Lewy Body Dementia Association (LBDA) is one of the leading resources for sufferers of DLB and their families. The LBDA features informational articles, support groups, an active community, and ways to help support the ongoing research of DLB. The LBDA has a website at http://www.lbda.org that offers all of these resources quickly wherever you can access the Internet. The LBDA also performs advocacy services for DLB sufferers, such as recently being involved in making disability claims for DLB easier to achieve.

The LBDA site has resources to help find support groups in your local area. If you go to http://www.lbda.org/content/local-lbd-support-groups, you can search for local groups by state. The Internet can be a great source of information and support, but sometimes having an actual, physical person to associate with can make much more impact than words on a screen. Elderly DLB sufferers might also suffer from an inability to operate a computer efficiently due to Parkinsonism or cognitive impairment. Seeking local help is usually a quick and painless process, and there is no harm in looking. These groups can also help coordinate resources and make dealing with the financial, emotional, and time costs of care-giving easier.

For those in the European area, http://www.lewybody.org/ is the site of the Lewy Body Society. The LBS is similar to the LBDA in its support of research and providing information and resources about DLB. The Lewy Body Foundation is a smaller non-profit organization centered in Australia that supports independent research of DLB. They can be found online at http://lewybodyfoundation.wordpress.com/.

Many have opted to share their personal stories with others online, such as the Lewy Body Journal at http://www.lewybodyjournal.org/. The Journal is a recording of one family's experience when the mother was diagnosed with DLB in 1996, until her death in May 2006. The site continues to update with information to this day. There is also an active Yahoo! Message board group centered on DLB caregivers at http://health.groups.yahoo.com/group/LBDcaregivers/.

The Right Treatment for You

There is no such thing as one right answer with a disease as complicated as Lewy Body Dementia. The treatment options listed here are not all of the options available, but the information should give a good start in finding the right medicinal and therapy treatments for you or your loved one. As with any advice on medical subjects, be sure to consult with your primary care physician before acting on any information, and never hesitate to ask for second opinions when you feel you need them. The entire process should be about finding the right treatment options for you or your loved one.

How to Care for a Relative with Lewy Body Dementia

When you choose to care for a person with Lewy Body Dementia (LBD), you must expect some hard times, but also rewarding moments that can deepen the relationship between you and your loved one. You should take a proactive approach to the disease and learn as much as you can about it, since this will greatly increase the effectiveness of your care. If you are well informed, you will know how LBD is likely to affect your loved one specifically.

How Do I Tell My Loved One About His or Her Condition?

One important decision is whether to tell the affected person about his or her condition. Most experts agree that they should be told of their diagnosis, but also remark that the extent of details and the timing of the discussion are essential to get a good reaction. If the person is troubled by the symptoms already experienced, it is probably a good idea not to delay the news. It often happens that the patient becomes frustrated by the things she cannot do anymore, wondering what is wrong. In those cases, you should be fair to your loved one and explain the situation in a mature way. If you do not acknowledge the experiences he or she is having, your loved one will probably feel more frustrated and worried.

The reaction might be more positive than we expect. An article in the Journal of the American Geriatrics Society stated that, "disclosure of a dementia diagnosis does not prompt a catastrophic emotional reaction in most people, even those who are only mildly impaired, and may provide some relief once an explanation for symptoms is known and a treatment plan is developed." One caretaker also stated: "My father's reaction wasn't nearly as terrible as I had feared. It almost seemed to me that he was somewhat relieved to know that he wasn't having funny thoughts."

Once you disclose the news, you must carefully watch the reaction of your loved one. Some people may deny suffering dementia, but they may acknowledge their memory is failing. If that is the case, it is probably wise to use the words "memory loss" when communicating with them, rather than "dementia." It is possible that your loved one will deny the condition altogether. Should that happen you need to be patient, since it can be a defense mechanism or a symptom of the illness. Their attitude will probably change after some time has passed.

You must bear in mind that many affected people are not aware of the limitations dementia imposes on them, or they might simply forget the symptoms. Every person is different, and in some cases you will be able to speak freely with your loved one about his condition. With others it will be best just to take care of them, without going into the dynamics or root causes and effects of the illness.

What Kind of Specialist Should Treat an LBD Patient?

There are several kinds of professionals trained to evaluate and treat the symptoms, such as geriatricians, geriatric psychiatrists and neurologists. Since there is not really a specific medical branch specialized in dementia, the best course of action is looking for a physician with ample experience in this kind of disease, more specifically with memory disorders. If you contact your local or national Alzheimer's Association, they will likely be able to advice you, since LBD's symptoms are very similar to Alzheimer's. You can also call your medical insurer or hospital and ask them to recommend a specialized physician, who will typically belong to one of the aforementioned disciplines.

Dealing with Sleep Problems

Lack of proper sleep is one of the main problems for people with LBD. In fact, many of the patients who end up in nursing homes do so for this reason. Sleeping disorders can be caused to alcohol use, medications, stress, bad sleep habits or an additional illness. There could also be underlying sleeping difficulties undetected prior to dementia. One particular problem is "sun downing", which consists of a period of increased confusion and restlessness, beginning at dusk and continuing all night. In the worst case, this will make proper sleep impossible for your loved one, causing drowsiness the next day. There are several measures you can take to prevent agitation during the night. Here are some of them:

* Keep alcohol away from your loved one

Alcohol consumption can increase confusion and botch their senses even more, so serving alcohol to the person under your care is a very bad idea. If they insist on having it, try giving them a soft drink in a cocktail glass, or give them non-alcoholic beer or wine. If it is late in the day, you should also avoid serving your loved one any beverage containing caffeine, such as black tea, cola drinks and coffee, since it will likely disrupt his or her sleep.

* Plan activities and exercises for your loved one

You must find a balance that allows keeping your loved one under your care active, but without causing exhaustion. Walks, car and bicycle rides will help your loved one to use his energy effectively while helping him to sleep well in the night. These exercises will also improve his health and spirit, and will reinforce his sense of routine. Always remember to decrease the intensity of the activities as the dusk approaches and also avoid overstimulation, since it will likely lead to exhaustion.

* Establish set times of sleep

It is important not to deviate from specific times of sleeping, since that will likely lead to restlessness. Ideally, these times should be as approximate as possible to the ones the person had during his active years. Although the most important goal is to get your loved one to sleep well, oversleeping should not be encouraged. Therefore, you should be mindful of the waking up time too.

* Limit naps

Your loved one might need a nap, typically after lunch. If that is the case, make sure it is short, since that will likely disrupt his or her sleep during the night. These naps should be taken in a couch or similar furniture, so the person does not associate the bed to night time sleep. You must also try to avoid naps late in the day.

* Establish bedtime routines

For instance, you can listen to relaxing music or give your loved one a back-rub, following the same pattern every day, including the use of the bathroom. As with the other routines, this will comfort the person under your care and help his sleep. If putting on night clothes is difficult for your loved one, it should be done earlier in the day, to avoid unnecessary stress near bedtime.

* Make sleeping comfortable

The bedroom should be a quiet and relaxing place. Make sure there are a number of familiar objects around, since they will help a great deal. If your loved one has a favorite blanket, try to have it always available. The person's bed clothes must be as comfortable and unrestrictive as possible. It is usually a good idea to have a night light turned on. The path to the bathroom must also be clear of obstacles and sufficiently lit.

*Be gentle on your loved one when she starts giving you trouble in the night.

Some people with LBD awaken during the night and show unrest. In such an instance, ask them what they need and reassure them. Don't scold your loved one, since it will only make things worse. Announce that it is sleep time to help them become aware of the situation. If your loved one has gotten out of the bedroom, gently guide her back and do what is needed in order to have her sleep again. You could adopt the style of repeating bedtime rituals or speaking to her gently.

* Seek assistance from a doctor

Some sleep problems can be caused by ailments such as incontinence or an underlying sleep disorder, like apnea. Have your loved one examined by a doctor, who will be able to diagnose if something's wrong and prescribe the right treatment or medication if needed. Sometimes it may be necessary to change the medication of your loved one. This could also be determined by the doctor. Bedtime can be a tough trial, especially during the first few months. One caretaker said "For me it was the hardest part, since I still had to wake up early to go to work every day, it was like having babies all over again. Nevertheless, you end up adapting, just like when you are a parent. My wife was wonderful and took turns with me to check out on my father."

Some Basic Caretaking Tips

Apart from learning how to deal with sleep problems of your loved one, here are some basic caretaking tips you should know:

* Create routines

It often helps persons with Lewy Body Dementia to have daily routines, especially concerning their meal and sleep times. They will help them to feel safer and to organize their day. Assigning light housekeeping chores to your loved one is also a good idea, since it can reduce the restlessness which often leads to agitation or aggression. You should always try to keep the routine and environment of your loved one consistent and simple. Any change can cause unrest, so if you absolutely need to do it, you should do it gradually.

* Minimize risks

People with LBD are often prone to falls. To help minimize this risk, you should help your loved one stabilize his blood pressure, making sure he stands up slowly; stays well hydrated; takes in an adequate amount of salt; and does not overstay in bed. A doctor should also examine the five senses of your loved one and treat any abnormalities or advice specific exercises. If the person under your care walks with a shuffle, provide a cane or walker, which will add support and confidence. Walkers are often met with resistance, but will probably reduce the risk of falls more than a cane. You will need to remind your loved one to use his walking aid, as he might forget he has to. Make sure he is in clear view. You can also reduce risks by removing throw rugs and clutter usually found in pathways.

* Make things easy

When giving tasks to your loved one to keep her active or in shape, they should be broken into easy steps. Remember to praise successes and minimize failures. It is not advisable to teach her new information or ask her to perform tasks she couldn't complete in the past, since it will only result in frustration. You should not test their memory either. If you need to ask your loved one a question, make it easy to understand and ask one at a time. Try to always behave pleasantly. You might be feeling stressed or angry, but you must not let it show. Speak to your loved one in a calm way, and if he or she feels unrest due to failure, give him or her reassurance and distract her with some other activity.

* Prevent aggressive reactions

As stated, it is not atypical for patients with any kind of dementia to become anxious, frustrated or unable to communicate, which can lead to an angry behavior. They also may have a catastrophic reaction (in other words, an emotional outburst) to a variety of events, such as loud noises from radio, TV or people, multiple or difficult questions (like those including the concept "why"), small accidents, reprimands, a feeling of being left out, a tense caregiver, etc. When your loved one becomes aggressive, the golden rule is to always stay calm and talk to him till he returns to a peaceful state. There are other actions that can trigger aggressiveness, such as laughing or whispering, that can easily be misinterpreted by people with Lewy Body Dementia, so it is best to avoid them as much as possible. In other cases, anxiety can be caused by some form of physical pain, so be sure to regularly consult with a doctor to make sure nothing is bothering them. One caretaker said about this: "After the first few months I learned a lot of self control, and my own calmness soon reflected on my mother's. It was much easier from then on."

Getting Home Care and Rest

Caregiving for dementia patients can be overwhelming and time-demanding. If you and your family feel you are not able to do it by yourselves, it is a good idea to enlist external help. You can choose among a number of options, from volunteers to paid caregivers. Carefully consider which one best suits your needs and those of your loved one, as well as your economic ability. You might need only short breaks or permanent help of varying degrees. You must be aware that it can take some time to get this help, so plan in advance. Here are some options to consider:

Volunteers: Check for associations and churches in your area that do social volunteering work. Volunteers can help in simple tasks such as giving companionship, running errands or cooking. But they might be willing to give more help, just ask them. There are also healthy people of advanced age who enjoy taking care of others who haven't been so lucky.

Homemakers: They can help with house chores such as cleaning, grocery shopping, cooking and laundry. Although this isn't complete caretaking, if they help you with these tasks, you will be able to devote more time to the person under your care with greater attention.

Personal attendants and nurses: This is the most involved kind of assistance. Personal attendants will help with personal care tasks such as bathing and dressing. Most often, they will have to be paid for their services. If you need this kind of assistance, first check what your loved one's insurance covers. You can also contact an attorney in order to determine what your state allows for assistance of elderly people. Your loved one might qualify for an aid program.

In order to find the best person to help you, it is a great idea to make a list of questions for the candidates. Here are some suggested questions you could ask:

* What is your training?

* Have you got some prior experience with these kinds of patients?

* Why have you chosen this line of work?

* Do you have any special abilities that might help?

One very important question to ask is what they would do in hypothetical situations that might happen to the person they are caring for, such as what they would do if the patient is falling down or straying away from home. Their response to such a question will give you a better idea of their capabilities. Also, you should check their references.

You might have some reservations about putting your loved one under the care of others, but if you carefully choose the person, it will end up being a great help and relief for you, especially if you're tight on time and have other obligations. The hired caretaker can develop strong bonds with the family. "I don't know what I'd have done without her, I could tell she really cared for dad, and strangely enough, due to his memory problems, he ended up considering her family," said the daughter of a LBD patient about her hired assistant.

The Caregiver Must also be Cared For

It is of extreme importance that you as a caregiver also take care of yourself. There are some important measures that will help you to cope with the situation and maintain a good physical and mental state. Here are some of them:

Take breaks: You can't devote all your time to the person with LBD, so be sure to rest every once in a while and if possible, get out of the house and do some leisure activities.

Do exercises daily: This is important not only because being in good shape will help with your caregiving tasks, but because exercise is very good for the mind too. If you can't exercise for a long period of time due to your obligations, do it in short sessions.

Keep seeing your friends and relatives: Don't neglect your friends and family, since hanging out with them is good by itself, but often they also offer selfless help.

Communicate with people in similar situations: It is a great idea to share your experiences with people who are also taking care of a person with LBD. You can do this either in person or through Internet forums and chats. You'll soon see that others can give you great relief and advice, and that you can do the same thing. Good advice can help you in your caregiving and coping, so share your knowledge and learn from others. You might also be interested in joining an LBD-related association.

Have fun with your loved one: Even when the person you are taking care of is not at the peak of his or her abilities, you can have great times with them, just by taking walks, playing easy and fun games or stroking a pet. You'll be surprised how much you can still enjoy life together. "It's not really about how much a person knows or remembers, but how they feel about you, that you are there almost to the very end. When I walked hand by hand with my mother, it was almost exactly like in the old days", said the daughter of an LBD patient about their regular strolls.

Symptoms during the Final Stages

As the illness advances, there's a severe cognitive decline, with the patient occasionally forgetting the name of their friends and relatives, or even of the person who takes care of them all the time, though they'll recall their own name in almost all cases. Despite forgetting names, they'll frequently continue distinguishing familiar from unfamiliar persons. For the most part, they won't remember recent events of their lives, having some knowledge of their past, but usually very sketchy. Generally, they won't be aware of their surroundings or the time of the year, and may also have difficulties with tasks like counting to 10. They will require assistance for most activities, and may become incontinent. They'll also find it hard moving around, but may manage by themselves if they're in familiar surroundings. They may exhibit delusional behavior, like accusing their spouse of being an impostor, talking to imaginary figures or to their reflection in the mirror. They may also have obsessive behaviors, like continually repeating simple cleaning activities. Anxiety and agitation also become frequent in the behavior.

At the very last stages, the person becomes profoundly demented and loses mobility. They will become weaker, gradually lose weight and become more susceptible to respiratory infections and similar ailments. At this stage their physical health is extremely delicate, so they can pass away due to pneumonia or some other illness. Due to the loss of strength, they won't be able to sit up on bed or hold up their heads without help. Eventually they won't be able to talk, will be sleeping most of the time, won't know anyone and will have to be hand fed. They will usually find it difficult to chew and swallow, so nutrition ends up being a problem. When oral feeding becomes impossible, it is time for the specialized doctor to decide if your loved one to be fed intravenously. Many people choose not to do so, since they feel that at that point it's meaningless, and therefore instruct the doctors to give only palliative care.

Fluctuating Cognition

Fluctuating cognition refers to the levels of awareness of the patient over a certain time interval. This symptom is specific to Lewy Body Dementia (LBD) and it is commonly used to identify whether the patient is suffering from LBD, as it is not common in Alzheimer's. At times, people who are suffering from LBD may appear much better than they actually are. Nevertheless, the intervals where the patient seems alert and in her right state of mind don't last long and there will be an observable downward progression after a couple of months.

Fluctuating behavior actually starts off with occasional moments when the patient acts oddly. With the passage of time, the confused behavior that is common to patients with dementia will appear more frequently, although there will be times when the patient will appear to behave normally. The spikes of awareness that LBD patients undergo can differ from one person to another and caregivers who sit down with patients and monitor their progress classify fluctuations into three categories: show times, bad times and good times.

Show Times

Every person has the innate desire to impress and this is also applicable to LBD patients. When someone they love or someone important comes to visit them, they act as if they are better than they actually are. Since LBD patients do not have impulse control, they do not choose to act as if they are normal. Show times happen because of the ingrained impulse to impress. However, this is very taxing to the patient as illustrated by the following case:

Marion, whose mother suffered from LBD, observed that every time they take a trip to the doctor's office, her mom would walk up straighter than she does at home. She also talked better and her answers made sense. However, when they leave, she'd slump again and just sleep on the next day.

Bad Times

This is the period in which the patient becomes confused about reality. At first, these confusing moments only happen in passing, but since dementia is degenerative, these hazes last longer and longer and this isolated behavior ultimately becomes the norm. Howard, whose wife has LBD, observes that in place of his extrovert and sociable wife is an old woman who is demanding, irrational and very possessive. She gets jealous of anyone who visits and she wants to know where he is all the time.

Good Times

The biggest difference between LBD and Alzheimer's disease is the fact that patients with LBD have windows of awareness. Although the patient experiences fewer periods of normalcy as their dementia worsens, these moments are really valued by caregivers and family members alike.

During these good times, it would be best to ask important questions to the patient and share moments together. Jenny made use of his husband's good times to ask for his approval to sell their car. Since he was fully aware during that time, he didn't make a fuss later.

Keeping track of these good times is very important since this can make life easier for caregivers. Family members and loved ones can also utilize such time to include the patient in making important life or treatment decisions.

Hospice Care

Hospice is a place of care for the terminally ill where treatment is focused on relieving and preventing the suffering of the patient (palliative treatment). When a person with LBD is given a prognosis of six months or less to live, the patient is eligible for hospice care, so she can receive the best palliative treatment. However, there is no way to know how long that person will live, since in some cases the decline is very slow, so it might still be possible to take care of the person in the home. Your loved one will remain eligible for hospice care if he or she has a measurable decline from one month to the other and her prognosis can be re-certified by the physician.

Hospices usually have accessibility agreements with local nursing homes. So if you take a patient to a nursing home that does not have a contract with a particular hospice, you can start one at any given moment. The nursing home can also contact a hospice on your behalf. Once the person with Lewy Body Dementia starts receiving hospice care, an entire team of professionals will go there to help with the particular symptoms of the disease. The hospice nurse will determine if there is a need to give special training to the facility staff. In the final stages of a person suffering from LBD, hospice care is probably the best option. But while you leave your loved one under hospice care, it will be important to visit with him frequently, since familiar faces will generally ease his stress and comfort him.

Finally, be informed that after diagnosis of Lewy Body Dementia, the average rate of survival is about seven years, though some people live much longer. But with proper care, those years can be meaningful for both you and your loved one.

Legal and Financial Issues in Lewy Body Dementia

LBD's incurability and progressive nature mean it will be a constant issue that can take tolls on the sufferer and their family. Apart from the pain of watching a loved one suffer with dementia, there are matters of legal and financial management that do not go away because you are dealing with hardship. Seeking help in financial and legal matters is essential, even if it is just to ask for advice on how to properly deal with them.

As LBD progresses, legal issues regarding guardianship, estate management, and care will continue to arise. It is important to be prepared for these issues with both educating yourself and seeking professional legal advice. The specifics of law vary state to state, and finding a local and reputable attorney to help make sure proper care is taken of these legal matters is essential. Do not attempt to go without an attorney, as one overlooked form or document can mean disaster in the legal world.

Progression of dementia can result in an eventual classification of a person as being incapable of caring for themselves, and needing a guardian. Most people are familiar with a power of attorney, but in the case of someone being declared mentally incompetent most normal powers of attorney will not function any more. Many attorneys with experience in dealing with dementia will recommend a version called a durable power of attorney that can last through declarations of incompetence.

Separate powers will be necessary for medical care, financial matters, and legal matters. It is important for both the sufferer to know they will be in the care of someone who has their best wishes at heart if the dementia progresses, and for caregivers to know they can give the care their loved ones deserve. Attorneys can help make stipulations on when these powers come into effect, which can be a level of assurance for sufferers from the thought of their rights to decide for themselves being taken away without cause.

The cost of legal service can be a deterrent from many people seeking help. Attorney fees are just one of the many financial problems that surface. If the sufferer was once a primary income earner in the household, the reduction to disability payments can be a dramatic difference from what they once earned. Medical bills can take a toll on what remains without expensive insurance that still might not cover all the costs. The time a caregiver needs to spend with their loved one can reduce the time they have available to work and generate more income.

There are resources available to help find legal advice when it is not possible to afford one on your own. Eldercare can help find attorneys with a focus in elder law who will work pro bono. The Agency of Aging office in your local area can also provide contacts, as can online support groups of families going through LBD. Many attorneys in these fields are familiar with the financial difficulties going through a persistent disease can place on a family, and are willing to do everything they can to help without placing more hardship on you.

Local support groups and organizations like the LBDA are also an option when financial difficulties become too much to bear altogether. They can help direct you to opportunities for assistance, help in getting Medicaid, and help manage daily needs like food and shelter. Many of these people will help purely from being in a position of having the capability. There is no shame in asking for help dealing with a disease that places an enormous amount of hardship on a family in more ways than just financially.

Organizations, Resources and Further Reading

Lewy Body Dementia Association

912 Killian Hill Road, S.W.

Lilburn, GA 30047

lbda@lbda.org

http://www.lbda.org

Tel: Telephone: 404-935-6444 Helpline: 800-539-9767

Fax: 480-422-5434

Alzheimer's Disease Education and Referral Center

(ADEAR)

National Institute on Aging (NIA)

P.O. Box 8250

Silver Spring, MD 20907-8250

adear@nia.nih.gov

http://www.nia.nih.gov/alzheimers

Tel: 301-495-3311 800-438-4380

Fax: 301-495-3334

Alzheimer's Association

225 North Michigan Avenue

Floor 17

Chicago, IL 60601-7633

info@alz.org

http://www.alz.org

Tel: 312-335-8700 1-800-272-3900 (24-hour helpline)
TDD: 312-335-5886

Fax: 866.699.1246

Family Caregiver Alliance/ National Center on
Caregiving

180 Montgomery Street

Suite 900

San Francisco, CA 94104

info@caregiver.org

http://www.caregiver.org

Tel: 415-434-3388 800-445-8106

Fax: 415-434-3508

Internet Resources / Further Reading

Merck Manual of Geriatrics

http://www.merck.com/mkgr/mmg/home.jsp

Similar in format to the Merck Manual of Diagnosis and Therapy, this guide focuses on disorders and diseases with a slant towards implications for the elderly.

Deciphering Medspeak

http://mlanet.org/resources/medspeak/index.html

To make informed health decisions, you have probably read a newspaper or magazine article, tuned into a radio or television program, or searched the Internet to find answers to health questions. If so, you have probably encountered "medspeak," the specialized language of health professionals. The Medical Library Association developed "Deciphering Medspeak" to help translate common "medspeak" terms.

National Center for Complementary and Alternative Medicine

http://nccam.nih.gov/

General information about alternative and complementary therapies with links to research studies currently being conducted on alternative therapies for a variety of conditions.

Clinical Research Trials

Center Watch

http://www.centerwatch.com/

Information on over 41,000 clinical trials for twenty disease categories. Profiles of 150 research centers conducting clinical trials and profiles of companies that provide a variety of contract services to the clinical trials industry. Includes industry and government sponsored clinical trials and information on new drug treatments approved by the Food and Drug Administration.

Clinical Trials

http://www.clinicaltrials.gov/

Information on current research being conducted on treatments for different diseases. Browse by disease category and sponsor or search the entire site. Learn what clinical trials are all about and how to decide to participate in a trial.

Health Care Providers

American Board of Medical Specialties (ABMS)

http://www.abms.org/

Verify the certification status of any physician in the 24 specialities of the ABMS. Registration is required (free) and user is limited to five searches in a 24 hour period.

AMA Physician Select

https://extapps.ama-assn.org/doctorfinder/recaptcha.jsp

Gives credentials of MD's and DO's including medical school, year of graduation, and specialties.

Federation of State Medical Boards

http://www.fsmb.org/

Select "Public Services" from the left-hand index, then select "Directory of State Medical Boards" to find links to web sites for the 50 U.S. States, plus the District of Columbia, Guam, and the Northern Mariana Islands. Not all of the states have physician profile or disciplinary action information. There are also links to osteopathic physician sites when available.

Nursing Home Compare

http://www.medicare.gov/NHCompare/Include/DataSection/Questions/SearchCriteriaNEW.asp?version=default&browser=Chrome|6|WinNT&language=English&defaultstatus=0&pagelist=Home&CookiesEnabledStatus=True

Provides detailed information about the performance of every Medicare and Medicaid certified nursing home in the country. Searchable by state. Includes a guide to choosing a nursing home and a nursing home checklist to help in making informed choices.

Quackery and Health Fraud

Quackwatch

http://www.quackwatch.com/

Want information about whether those alternative therapies work? This site has information on health fraud, medical quackery, "new age" medicine and "alternative" and "complementary" medicine.

National Council against Health Fraud

http://www.ncahf.org/

Non-profit voluntary health agency focusing on health fraud, misinformation, and quackery as public health oncerns. Read their position papers on acupuncture, homepathy, chiropractic, and other health issues.

Local Dementia with Lewy Bodies Support Groups

(In state order)

Mat-Su Area—Alzheimer's and Related Dementias Caregiver's Support Group
Meeting Dates and Times: Second Wednesday of every month, 1:00 p.m. – 2:30 p.m.
Who: For caregivers, friends, and family of those diagnosed with Dementia with Lewy bodiess, Alzheimer's disease and related dementias.
Where: Mile 2.2 Palmer-Wasilla Hwy at the Trinity Barn Plaza; Palmer, AK 99645
Who to Contact:
Sam Meneses
907.746.3413
SMeneses@alzalaska.org

Johns Island Dementia Caregiver Support Group
Meeting Dates and Times: Third Thursday of every month, 1 p.m. – 2 p.m.

Who: Caregivers, family members, friends, and health care professionals, in the Greater Charleston/Tri-county area caring for persons with progressive forms of dementia from diseases such as Dementia with Lewy bodies, Alzheimer's disease, Pick's disease, vascular dementia, frontotemperal dementia, or Parkinson's disease.
Where: Episcopal Church of Our Saviour
Address: 4416 Betsy Kerrison Parkway Johns Island, AL 29455
Who to Contact:
Laura Stefanelli
843.478.8756
laurastef@comcast.net

Morgan County Alabama Alzheimer's Disease and Related Dementia Support Group
Meeting Dates and Times: Third Tuesday of every month, 7:00 p.m. – 8:30 p.m.
Who: Caregivers, family and friends of those with dementia related diseases, including those with LBD.
Where: Mental Health Association in Morgan County
Address: 207 Commerce Circle SW Decatur, AL 35601
Who to Contact:
Nina Mae Blackburn
256.353.1160
ninablackburn@mhainmc.net

East Valley Dementia with Lewy bodies Support Group
Meeting Dates and Times: Fourth Thursday of every month, 1:00pm -3:00 p.m.
Who: Caregivers and family members of those diagnosed with Dementia with Lewy bodies.
Where: Arbor Rose Senior Care
Address: 6033 East Arbor Avenue Mesa, AZ 85206
Who to Contact:

Marla J. Burns
480.641.2531
mjblbdaz@gmail.com

Bay Area - Dementia with Lewy bodies Caregiver Support Group

Meeting Dates and Times: Approximately every six weeks on a Sunday, 5 p.m. – 7 p.m. (call for date information)
Who: Caregivers of those with Dementia with Lewy bodies.
Where: Mimi's Cafe
Address: Where: 2208 Bridgepointe Parkway San Mateo, CA 94404
Who to Contact:
Robin Riddle
650.814.0848
rriddle@stanfordalumni.org

Gold River Lewy Body Support Group

Meeting Dates and Times: Second Thursday of every month, 10 a.m. – 11:30 a.m.
Who: Caregivers and loved ones of those diagnosed with Dementia with Lewy bodies.
Where: Eskaton Lodge Gold River, Assisted Living and Memory Care
Address: 11390 Coloma Road Gold River, CA 95670
Who to Contact:
Denise Davis
916.930.9080
denise.davis@alznorcal.org

High Desert Dementia with Lewy bodies Support Group

Meeting Dates and Times: Who to Contact Stephanie Brynjolfson for details.
Who: For caregivers and family members of those diagnosed with Dementia with Lewy bodies.
Where: Who to Contact Stephanie Brynjolfson for details.

Address: Who to Contact Stephanie Brynjolfson for details. Who to Contact Stephanie Brynjolfson for details., CA 99999
Who to Contact:
Stephanie Brynjolfson
760.963.1478
stephanieinga@hotmail.com

Irvine/Alzheimer's Association Caregiver Support Group
Meeting Dates and Times: Second Tuesday of every month, 1:00 p.m. – 2:30 p.m.
Who: Dementia with Lewy bodies and frontotemporal dementia caregivers.
Where: Alzheimer's Association
Address: 17771 Cowan Street., Suite 290 Irvine, CA 92614
Who to Contact:
Donna Velarde
949.757.3759
donna.velarde@alz.org

Irvine/UCI Caregiver Support Group
Meeting Dates and Times: First Wednesday of every month, 9:30 a.m. – 11:30 a.m. (RSVP recommended for parking permits)
Who: Dementia with Lewy bodies and fronto-temporal dementia caregivers.
Where: University of California-Irvine campus, Gillespie Neuroscience Research Facility, first floor conference room
Address: University of California-Irvine campus, Gillespie Neuroscience Research Facility, first floor conference room Irvine, CA 99999
Who to Contact:
Susan Randhawa, MSW
949.824.2983
susanr@uci.edu

North Bay Dementia with Lewy bodies Support Group

Meeting Dates and Times: Second Tuesday of every month 4:30 p.m. – 6:00 p.m.
Who: Caregivers and family members who have a loved one with Dementia with Lewy bodies.
Where: The Atrium Court building
Address: 1260 North Dutton Avenue, 1st floor conference room - #140 Santa Rosa, CA 95401
Who to Contact:
Laurie White
707.525.9633
laurie@dementiaconsulting.com

Northern California/East Bay LBD and other Dementias Support Group
Meeting Dates and Times: Second Tuesday of every month from 7:15 p.m. to 9:00 p.m. in the Community Meeting Room.
Who: Family members who have a loved one with Dementia with Lewy bodies, or any other dementia.
Where: Robert Livermore Community Center
Address: 4444 East Avenue Livermore, CA 94550
Who to Contact:
Karen Jenkins
925.325.0544
kjenkins@rsac.com

Palm Desert Area Alzheimer's Family Support Group
Meeting Dates and Times: Every Thursday, 9:00 a.m. – 11:00 a.m.
Who: Family members who have a loved one with Alzheimer's disease, Dementia with Lewy bodies, or any other dementia.
Where: Eisenhower Medical Center Five Star Club
Address: Beacon Hill, Suite A Palm Desert, CA 92211
Who to Contact:

Stacy Smith
760.836.0232
ssmith@emc.org

Sacramento Pocket Area Dementia with Lewy bodies Support Group
Meeting Dates and Times: Fourth Wednesday of every month, 2:30 p.m. – 4:30 p.m.
Who: Caregivers, and loved ones of those diagnosed with Dementia with Lewy bodies.
Where: Primrose Specialized Senior Living
Address: 7707 Rush River Drive Sacramento, CA 95831
Who to Contact:
Kim Winters BSG., M.Ed
916.392.3510
kow@primrosealz.com

San Diego County Dementia with Lewy bodies and Frontotemporal Dementia Caregiver Support Group
Meeting Dates and Times: First Wednesday of every month, 2:00 p.m. – 3:30 p.m.
Who: For Dementia with Lewy bodies and fronto-temporal dementia caregivers.
Where: Shiley-Marcos UCSD Alzheimer's Disease Research Center Conference Room
Address: 8950 Villa La Jolla Drive, Suite C-129 La Jolla, CA 92037
Who to Contact:
Lisa Snyder
858.622.5800
lsnyder@AD.UCSD.EDU

Santa Ynez Valley Caregivers Support Group
Meeting Dates and Times: First and third Tuesday of every month, 2:00 p.m. - 3:30 p.m.

Who: For caregivers and family members who have a loved one with Dementia with Lewy bodies, Alzheimer's disease, or any other dementia.
Where: Solvang Friendship House, Hamilton Room
Address: 880 Friendship Lane Solvang, CA 93463
Who to Contact:
Ari Weaver
805.688.5868
smithweaver@yahoo.com

Colorado Springs Dementia with Lewy bodies Support Group
Meeting Dates and Times: First Monday of every month, 10:00 a.m. – 12:00 p.m.
Who: Caregivers and family members of loved ones with LBD.
Where: St. Francis Hospital, Conference Room 5
Address: 6001 East Woodmen Road Colorado Springs, CO 80923
Who to Contact:
Marika Flynn
719.440.7863
mudflynn@yahoo.com

Metro Denver Dementia Caregivers Support Group
Meeting Dates and Times: The first Thursday of each month, 6:30 p.m. - 8:30 p.m.
Who: For those who care for people with dementia, including Dementia with Lewy bodies and Alzheimer's Disease
Where: Good Shepherd Episcopal Church (This church is located off I-25 and Dry Creek Road, just west of the Dry Creek/Yosemite intersection.)
Address: 8545 East Dry Creek Road Centennial, CO 80112
Who to Contact:

Deb Wells
303.549.1886
debkwells@comcast.net

Northern Colorado Dementia with Lewy bodies Support Group

Meeting Dates and Times: Second and fourth Saturday of every month, 9:30 a.m. to 11 a.m.
Who: For caregivers and family members of those diagnosed with LBD.
Where: Medical Center of the Rockies (Poudre Canyon Room)
Address: 2500 Rocky Mountain Avenue Loveland, CO 80538
Who to Contact:
Karen Waldron
970.219.0898 or 970.282.7183
keakw@comcast.net

Fairfield County/New Haven County Dementia with Lewy bodies Support Group

Meeting Dates and Times: Third Monday of every month 6:30 p.m. – 8:30 p.m.
Who: For caregivers and loved ones of those diagnosed with Dementia with Lewy bodies.
Where: Primary Care Physicians of Fairfield
Address: 111 Beach Road Fairfield, CT 06824
Who to Contact:
Kristen Cusato
760.420.7063
kcusato@yahoo.com
Margaret Ricker
203.259.7442 x12

Greater Hartford Lewy Body Support Group

Meeting Dates and Times: Third Tuesday of every month, 6:30 p.m. - 8:30 p.m.

Who: People who want support coping with Dementia with Lewy bodies, including caregivers, family members, health professionals and people living with LBD.
Where: West Hartford Senior Center
Address: 15 Starkel Road West Hartford, CT 06117
Who to Contact:
Amy Silverman
860.232.2452
amysilver123@comcast.net

Lower Fairfield County Dementia with Lewy bodies Support Group
Meeting Dates and Times: Third Tuesday of each month, 10:00am to 12:00pm
Who: Caregivers and family members of those diagnosed with Dementia with Lewy bodies.
Where: Atria Darien, Atria Senior Living Center
Address: 50 Ledge Road (exit 11 off I95) Darien, CT 06820
Who to Contact:
Lynne Gray
203.655.9966
lynnegray@hotmail.com

Delaware Valley Dementia with Lewy bodies Support Group
Meeting Dates and Times: Third Tuesday of every month, 6 p.m. – 7 p.m.
Who: Caregivers and loved ones of those with a Dementia with Lewy bodies diagnosis and who reside in Delaware, Pennsylvania, and New Jersey are welcome to attend.
Where: Rockland Place
Address: 1519 Rockland Road Wilmington, DE 19803
Who to Contact:
Erica Browning
302.299.7281
kempage@hotmail.com

East Central Florida Dementia with Lewy bodies Support Group
Meeting Dates and Times: Second Wednesday of every month, 10:00 am– 11:00am.
Who: For caregivers, friends, and family of those diagnosed with Dementia with Lewy bodiess
Where: Joe's Club
Address: 4676 Wickham Rd. Melbourne, FL 32935
Who to Contact:
DeAnn Collins
(321) 768-9575 ext. 6
DeAnn.Collins@Health-First.org

Highlands County Area Weekly Daytime Caregiver Support Group
Meeting Dates and Times: Every Thursday, 1 p.m. – 2 p.m.
Who: Family members of loved ones with progressive dementia.
Where: Sebring Christian Church
Address: 4514 Hammock Road Sebring, FL 33872
Who to Contact:
Jean Maas
863.314.9193
jeanmaas@embarqmail.com
Ellen McKissock
863.385.5408

Highlands County Area Weekly Evening Caregiver Support Group
Meeting Dates and Times: Every Thursday, 6:30 p.m. – 7:30 p.m.
Who: Family members of loved ones with progressive dementia.
Where: Sebring Christian Church
Address: 4514 Hammock Road Sebring, FL 33872
Who to Contact:

Jean Maas
863.314.9193
jeanmaas@embarqmail.com
Ellen McKissock
863.385.5408

Jacksonville, FL - Mayo Clinic Memory Disorder Clinic Alzheimer's and Related Dementia Education Series and Caregiver Support Group

Meeting Dates and Times: Third Tuesday of every month, 10:45 a.m. – noon.

Who: For family members to improve their understanding of dementia, including symptoms and behavior changes as well as understand the progression of the disease, plan for the future, and provide knowledge to assist in their caregiving role.

Where: Mayo Clinic Memory Disorder Clinic, Cannaday Building – Room 1106

Address: 4500 San Pablo Road Jacksonville, FL 32224

Who to Contact:

North Pinellas County Dementia with Lewy bodies Support Group

Meeting Dates and Times: Third Monday of every month, 6 p.m. to 7:30 p.m.

Who: Dementia with Lewy bodies caregivers and family members.

Where: Arden Courts Dementia Assisted Living (behind Manor Care)

Address: 2895 Tampa Road Palm Harbor, FL 34684

Who to Contact:
Debbie Langrock
727.784.6597 or 727.686.9272
dlangrock@preferhome.com

Pinellas County/Clearwater Dementia Caregiver Support Group

Meeting Dates and Times: Second and fourth Tuesdays of every month, 1:00 p.m.
Who: Dementia caregivers, including Dementia with Lewy bodies caregivers.
Where: Villas of Belleair (Assisted Living, Memory and Parkinson's Care Community
Address: 620 Belleair Road Clearwater, FL 33756
Who to Contact:
Rebecca Weitzel
727.467.9464 ext. 208
rww@villasob.com
Karen (Karle) Truman, Ph.D.
727.391.9999 Karen may be reached at this number on Mondays – Thursdays, 9 a.m. – 4 p.m.
karenkarle@knology.net

Pinellas County/Largo (daytime) Dementia Caregiver Support Group
Meeting Dates and Times: First and third Friday of every month, 9:30 a.m. – 11 a.m.
Who: Dementia caregivers, including Dementia with Lewy bodies caregivers.
Where: Grand Villa Assisted Living
Address: 750 Starkey Road Largo, FL 33771
Who to Contact:
Karen (Karle) Truman, Ph.D.
727.391.9999 on Mondays – Thursdays, 9 a.m. – 4 p.m.
karenkarle@knology.net

Pinellas County/Largo (evening) Dementia Caregiver Support Group
Meeting Dates and Times: First and third Tuesday of every month, 6 p.m. – 7:30 p.m.
Who: Dementia caregivers, including Dementia with Lewy bodies caregivers.
Where: Grand Villa Assisted Living
Address: 750 Starkey Road Largo, FL 33771

Who to Contact:
Karen (Karle) Truman, Ph.D.
727.391.9999 on Mondays - Thursdays, 9 a.m.- 4 p.m.
karenkarle@knology.net

Pinellas County/Palm Harbor Dementia Caregiver Support Group
Meeting Dates and Times: First and third Tuesday of every month, 9:30 a.m. – 11 a.m.
Who: Dementia caregivers, including Dementia with Lewy bodies caregivers.
Where: St. Mark Village Assisted Living
Address: 880 Highlands Blvd. Palm Harbor, FL 34684
Who to Contact:
Karen (Karle) Truman, Ph.D.
727.391.9999 on Mondays - Thursdays, 9 a.m.- 4 p.m.
karenkarle@knology.net

Polk County/Cypress Gardens Dementia Caregiver Support Group
Meeting Dates and Times: Fourth Wednesday of every month, 10 a.m. - 11:30 a.m.
Who: Dementia caregivers, including Dementia with Lewy bodies caregivers.
Where: The Meadows at Cypress Gardens
Address: 3050 Woodmont Avenue Winter Haven, FL 33884
Who to Contact:
Suzanne Lull
863.676.6000
suzcl63@gmail.com

Tampa Bay LBD Caregiver Support Group
Meeting Dates and Times: Second Monday of every month from 3:00 pm to 4:00 pm
Who: Caregivers and family members of those diagnosed with Dementia with Lewy bodies.
Where: USF Health Byrd Alzheimer's Center

Address: 4001 E. Fletcher Avenue Tampa, FL 33613
Who to Contact:
Nancy Teten, LCSW
(813) 974-6355
Andrea Dombrowski
(813) 974-6355
Betsy McDargh
813-486-1256
tampabaylewybodycaregivers@gmail.com

Atlanta Early Memory Loss Group/Class
Meeting Dates and Times: Fridays for 8 weeks, 10:30 a.m. - noon. Held twice a year in September-October and again in February-March.
Who: Open to people with mild cognitive impairment, early Alzheimer's disease, early LBD and early frontotemporal dementia. Couples are invited to participate where one person has been diagnosed with mild memory and cognitive changes. The group is divided so that the member of the couple who is experiencing memory or cognitive changes meets in one group and their spouse/care partner meets in another group. Single individuals experiencing early memory loss are also invited to participate in this group. They may come alone but are encouraged to bring a friend and/or family member to participate in the care partners group. Topics include: common changes in people faced with cognitive changes, role changes, memory aides, planning for the future and stress reduction.
Where: Emory Alzheimer's Disease Research Center
Address: 1841 Clifton Road Atlanta, GA 30329
Who to Contact:
Susan Peterson-Hazan, MSW, LCSW
404.728.6273
speter2@emory.edu

Caregiver Challenges Class: Everything A Caregiver Needs to Know about the Middle Stage of Dementia

Meeting Dates and Times: Fridays for 6 weeks, 10:30 a.m. – noon. Held twice a year in November-December and again in April-May.

Who: Class is designed to prepare caregivers for the middle stage of Alzheimer's disease, LBD, frontotemporal dementia and other neurodegenerative diseases. These progressive neurodegenerative diseases require families to plan for the future. Proactive planning can help ensure a high quality of life for the person with the illness as well as their family. Topics include: middle stage disease symptoms, behavior changes and strategies to cope with the changes, treatment options, legal planning issues, and resources to meet evolving needs.

Where: Emory Alzheimer's Disease Research Center
Address: 1841 Clifton Road Atlanta, GA 30329
Who to Contact:
Susan Peterson-Hazan, MSW, LCSW
404.728.6273
speter2@emory.edu

East Metro Atlanta Dementia with Lewy bodies Support Group
Meeting Dates and Times: Second Tuesday of every month, 10:00 a.m. – 12:00 p.m.
Who: For caregivers and family members of those diagnosed with Dementia with Lewy bodies.
Where: Merryvale Assisted Living Facility
Address: 11980 Highway 142 Oxford, GA 30054
Who to Contact:
Kathy Fowler
678.625.1899
kerf.lbda@gmail.com

Late Stage Dementia Class: Things A Caregiver Needs to Know about Late Stage Alzheimer's Disease, LBD and Frontotemporal Dementia

Meeting Dates and Times: Fridays for 4 weeks, 10:30 a.m. – noon. Held twice a year in January and again in May-June.
Who: Class is designed to prepare caregivers for the late and terminal stage of Alzheimer's disease, LBD, frontotemporal dementia and other neurodegenerative diseases. Topics to be covered include late stage physical symptoms of neurodegenerative diseases, ethical dilemma's that may occur and services available during the late stage, such as Hospice.
Where: Emory Alzheimer's Disease Research Center
Address: 1841 Clifton Road Atlanta, GA 30329
Who to Contact:
Susan Peterson-Hazan, MSW, LCSW
404.728.6273
speter2@emory.edu

IA/IL Quad Cities Dementia with Lewy bodies Support Group
Meeting Dates and Times: Third Tuesday of every month, 7:00 p.m. - 8:30 p.m.
Who: Caregivers and family members of those diagnosed with Dementia with Lewy bodies. Professionals working with LBD are also welcome.
Where: Trinity Hospital (in basement room A&B)
Address: 4500 Utica Ridge Road Bettendorf, IA 52722
Who to Contact:
Elizabeth Saelens
1.877.923.3890
info@srcare411.com

Fort Wayne Dementia with Lewy bodies Support Group
Meeting Dates and Times: Second Wednesday of every month, 7 p.m. - 8:15 p.m.
Who: For both caregivers and those diagnosed with LBD.
Where: Turnstone Center
Address: 3320 North Clinton Street Fort Wayne, IN 46805
Who to Contact:

Sarah Miller
260.580.6808
sarahmillerfbs@gmail.com

Kentuckiana Lewy Body and Related Dementias Support Group

Meeting Dates and Times: First Wednesday of every month, 11:00 a.m. – 12:00 p.m.
Who: Dementia caregivers, including Dementia with Lewy bodies caregivers.
Where: Arden Courts of Louisville (in the activities room)
Address: 10451 Linn Station Road Louisville, KY 40223
Who to Contact:
Angela Youngman
502.387.3898
angela.youngman@gmail.com

Dementia with Lewy bodies Support Group of the Bluegrass

Meeting Dates and Times: First Tuesday of each month from 6:00 p.m. - 8:00 p.m.
Who: Caregivers and loved ones of those diagnosed with Dementia with Lewy bodies
Where: Christ Church
Address: 3801 Harrodsburg Road Lexington, KY 40513
Who to Contact:
Daniel McIlwain
859-948-1660
lbdbluegrassky@gmail.com
Sue Dawson
928-853-8383
lbdbluegrassky@gmail.com

Northwest Louisiana Dementia with Lewy bodies Caregiver's Support Group

Meeting Dates and Times: Fourth Tuesday of every month, 2 p.m. – 3:30 p.m.

Who: Family and friends of people with LBD.
Where: Hospice of Shreveport/Bossier
Address: 3829 Gilbert Drive Shreveport, LA 71104
Who to Contact:
Grace Holcombe
800.824.4672
gragra02@att.net

Central Massachusetts LBD Caregivers Support Group
Meeting Dates and Times: First Wednesday of every month, 6:30 p.m. – 8:00 p.m.
Who: Caregivers and families of people diagnosed with Dementia with Lewy bodies.
Where: Southgate at Shrewsbury
Address: 30 Julio Drive Shrewsbury, MA 01545
Who to Contact:
Cathy Flanagan
508.735.2059
Catmandu117@aol.com

Metro Boston LBD Caregiver Support Group
Meeting Dates and Times: Second Thursday of every month, 6:00 p.m. – 7:30 p.m. (Please call to confirm the date and time.)
Who: For caregivers and family members of people diagnosed with Dementia with Lewy bodies.
Where: Grande Room at Sherrill House
Address: 135 South Huntington Avenue Jamaica Plain, MA 02130
Who to Contact:
Victoria Ruff
617.710.0136
octoryrose@yahoo.com

Norfolk County LBD Caregivers Support Group
Meeting Dates and Times: First Monday of every month, 6:30 p.m. - 8 p.m.

Who: For caregivers and family members of people diagnosed with Dementia with Lewy bodies.
Where: Who to Contact Kristin Orr for the meeting location.
Address: Who to Contact Kristin Orr for the meeting location. Who to Contact Kristin Orr for the meeting location., MA 99999
Who to Contact:
Kristin Orr
617.650.0717
southshoreLBD@gmail.com

North Shore Atypical Parkinson's Support Group
Meeting Dates and Times: Meets quarterly, 1:00 p.m. – 3:00 p.m. Who to Contact Ann Aversa for dates.
Who: People and families dealing with LBD, PSP, CBD, MSA and other similar neurological disease.
Where: Lahey Clinic Medical Center (Who to Contact Ann Aversa for information about the meeting room location at the Lahey Clinic.)
Address: 41 Mall Road Burlington, MA 01705
Who to Contact:
Ann Aversa
617.872.8356
bappsg@comcast.net

South Shore Atypical Parkinson's Support Group
Meeting Dates and Times: Meets every other month (September, November, January, March, June), 2:30 p.m. – 4:00 p.m. Who to Contact Allyson for exact dates.
Who: People and families dealing with LBD, PSP, CBD, MSA and other similar neurological disease.
Where: Braintree Rehabilitation Hospital
Address: 250 Pond Street, 2nd Floor Conference Room Braintree, MA 02184
Who to Contact:

Allyson Gormley LICSW
617.638.7747
allyson.gormley@bmc.org

Baltimore County LBD Caregiver Support Group
Meeting Dates and Times: Who to Contact Kathleen
Hadaway for details.
Who: Caregivers and family members of those diagnosed
with Dementia with Lewy bodies.
Where: Morningside House of Satyr Hill
Address: 8800 Old Harford Road Parkville, MD 21234
Who to Contact:
Kathleen Hadaway
443.802.0734
kathycake@verizon.net

Portland Area Atypical-Parkinson's Support Group
Meeting Dates and Times: Meets quarterly. Who to
Contact Janet Edmunson for dates and times.
Who: People and families dealing with LBD, PSP, CBD,
MSA and other similar neurological disease.
Where: Parkinson's Information & Referral Center At Maine
Health Learning Resource Center
Address: 5 Buckman Road, Suite 1A Falmouth, ME 04105
Who to Contact:
Janet Edmunson
207.799.4963
janet@janetedmunson.com
Barby Johnson
207.633.0881
rockyledges@yahoo.com

Ann Arbor/Detroit Area Dementia with Lewy bodies
Support Group
Meeting Dates and Times: Second Wednesday of every
month, 6:00 p.m. - 7:30 p.m.

Who: Caregivers, family members and friends of those diagnosed with Dementia with Lewy bodies.
Where: Providence Hospital Medical Building (behind the hospital)
Address: 22250 Providence Drive, 8th Floor –Room C Southfield, MI 48075
Who to Contact:
Audra Frye
248.943.0556
5642MKTG@hcr-manorcare.com

South Shore Parkinson-Plus Support Group
Meeting Dates and Times: Second Wednesday of every other month (September, November, January, March, June) 2:30 p.m. – 4:00 p.m.
Who: Caregivers, family members and friends of those diagnosed with Dementia with Lewy bodies.
Where: Waltonwood at Cherry Hill (an assisted living and dementia care facility)
Address: 42600 Cherry Hill Road Canton, MI 48188
Who to Contact:
Audra Frye
248.943.0556
5642MKTG@hcr-manorcare.com

Minnesota East Metro LBD Caregiver Support Group
Meeting Dates and Times: Third Monday of every month, usually at 6:30 p.m.
Who: Caregivers and family members of those facing a diagnosis of Dementia with Lewy bodies. We provide a comfortable and compassionate place to share experiences, support, and resources as we journey with our loved one through the many phases of this disease.
Where: Lakeview Commons of Maplewood
Address: 1200 Lakewood Dr. N. Maplewood, MN 55119
Who to Contact:

Directions and General Information
651-773-7150
Paula Biever
651-641-0130
paula.biever@gmail.com
Erik Biever
651-641-0130
ebiever@gmail.com

Princeton Area Caregivers Support Group

Meeting Dates and Times: First Tuesday of every month, 10:00 a.m. - 11:30 a.m.

Who: For caregivers and family members of those diagnosed with Dementia with Lewy bodies, Alzheimer's Disease, Parkinson's Disease, and other dementias or neuro-degenerative diseases. The support group also welcomes caregivers who have lost someone to these diseases, and who would like to share their experiences with support group members or who would like ongoing support for themselves.

Where: Elim Care and Rehab Center

Address: 701 1st Street Princeton, MN 55371

Who to Contact:
Carolyn Stabene
763.243.2170
cstabene@yahoo.com
Phyllis Sueverkruepp
763.389.3251

Roseau Alzheimer's/LBD Awareness and Support Group

Meeting Dates and Times: Second Wednesday of every month, 6:30 p.m. – 8:00 p.m.

Who: Caregivers and family members who have a loved one with Dementia with Lewy bodies, Alzheimer's disease, or any other dementia.

Where: Roseau Masonic Lodge

Address: 711 Second Avenue SE Roseau, MN 56751

Who to Contact:
Jill Wulff
218.425.7401
jill.wulff@alz.org

Southwest Metro Minneapolis Caregiver Support Group
Meeting Dates and Times: Second Monday of every month, 12:00 p.m. – 2:00 p.m.
Who: For families facing a diagnosis of LBD and health care professionals working with persons with LBD who want information and support.
Where: Gianna Homes
Address: 4605 Fairhills Road East Minnetonka, MN 55345
Who to Contact:
Anne Marie Hansen
952.988.0953
anne@giannahomes.org

Twin Cities Metro Area Atypical Parkinson's Disease Support Group
Meeting Dates and Times: Second Wednesday of every month, 1:00 p.m. – 3:00 p.m.
Who: Anyone diagnosed or caring for someone diagnosed with a Parkinson's disease spectrum disorder, including Dementia with Lewy bodies, progressive supranuclear palsy, and multiple systems atrophy.
Where: Struthers Parkinson's Center
Address: 6701 Country Club Drive Golden Valley, MN 55427
Who to Contact:
Joan Hlas
952.993.6650
Joan.Hlas@ParkNicollet.com

Twin Cities Metro Area Caregiver Support Group
Meeting Dates and Times: Second Thursday of every month, 1 p.m. – 3 p.m.

Who: Caregivers of those living with movement disorders, including Dementia with Lewy bodies, Parkinson's disease.
Where: Struthers Parkinson's Center
Address: 6701 Country Club Drive Golden Valley, MN 55427
Who to Contact:
Joan Hlas
952.993.6650
Joan.Hlas@ParkNicollet.com

Twin Cities Southeast Metro Caregiver Support Group
Meeting Dates and Times: Second Thursday of every month, 6:30 p.m. – 8:30 p.m.
Who: Caregivers and family members who have a loved one with Dementia with Lewy bodies, Alzheimer's disease, or any other dementia.
Where: Peaceful Mind Homes
Address: 3808 Blackhawk Ridge Place Eagan, MN 55122
Who to Contact:
Kam Aggarwal
651.538.4499
Kam@peacefulmindhomes.com

Warroad Community Support Group
Meeting Dates and Times: Third Thursday of every month, noon – 1:30 p.m.
Who: Caregivers and family members who have a loved one with Dementia with Lewy bodies, Alzheimer's disease, or any other dementia.
Where: Warroad Senior Living Center
Address: 1401 Lake Street Northwest Warroad, MN 56763
Who to Contact:
Jill Wulff
218.425.7401
jill.wulff@alz.org

Crystal Coast Dementia with Lewy bodies Support Group
Meeting Dates and Times: Second Monday of each month, 1:00 p.m. - 3:00 p.m.
Who: For caregivers and family members of those diagnosed with Dementia with Lewy bodies.
Where: Leon Mann Senior Center
Address: 3820 Galantis Drive Morehead City, NC 28557
Who to Contact:
Barbara Hutchinson
252.269.9748
bbhutch44@yahoo.com

Parkinson and Dementia with Lewy bodies Support Group of Wilmington
Meeting Dates and Times: Fourth Tuesday of every month, 1:30 p.m. – 3:30 p.m.
Who: For caregivers and family members of loved ones diagnosed with Parkinson's disease and Dementia with Lewy bodies.
Where: Wilmington Senior Center
Address: 2222 South College Road Wilmington, NC 28483
Who to Contact:
Dick Freund
910.686.2583
FreundDP@aol.com

Piedmont Triad Dementia with Lewy bodies Support Group
Meeting Dates and Times: Meets the Second Monday of the month, 7:00 pm - 8:00pm
Who: For caregivers and family members of loved ones diagnosed with Dementia with Lewy bodies.
Where: Brighton Gardens of Greensboro
Address: 1208 New Garden Road Greensboro, NC 27410
Who to Contact:

Anne Tubaugh
336.292.1239
LBDTriad@gmail.com

Metro Omaha LBD Caregiver's Support Group
Meeting Dates and Times: Third Tuesday of every month,
1:00 p.m. - 2:30 p.m.
Who: For caregivers and family members of people
diagnosed with Dementia with Lewy bodies.
Where: Millard Branch Omaha Public Library
Address: 13214 Westwood Lane Omaha, NE 68144
Who to Contact:
Ann Taylor
402-452-3952
Annt88@cox.net

Monadnock Parkinson's Support Group
Meeting Dates and Times: First Tuesday of every month,
2:00 p.m. – 4:00 pm.
Who: Anyone who has Parkinson-like symptoms or
Parkinson's disease and their caregivers.
Where: Saint James Episcopal Church's Undercroft on the
lower level
Address: 44 West Street Keene, NH 03431
Who to Contact:
Joe Nicholas
603.352.1727
jnicholas@ne.rr.com

Albuquerque Frontolobe Dementias Support Group
Meeting Dates and Times: First Sunday of every month,
2:00 p.m. - 5:30 p.m.
Who: For caregivers and family members of people
diagnosed with any type of Fronotolobe dementias.
Where: Who to Contact Gretchen Crowe for details.
Address: Who to Contact Gretchen Crowe for details.
Albuquerque, NM 87122

Who to Contact:
Gretchen Crowe
505-823-1554
ggshipley@comcast.net

Las Vegas Valley Dementia with Lewy bodies Support Group
Meeting Dates and Times: Fourth Thursday of every month, 5:00 p.m. – 6:00 p.m.
Who: For caregivers and family members of those diagnosed with Dementia with Lewy bodies.
Where: Adult Day Care Center of Las Vegas, Lied/Sinai Senior Care Campus
Address: 901 N Jones Blvd Las Vegas, NV 89108
Who to Contact:
Joan Croft
702.789.8371
LewyBodySupportLasVegas@hotmail.com

Long Island Area Support Group
Meeting Dates and Times: Fourth Monday of every month, 7:00 p.m – 8:30 p.m.
Who: Dementia with Lewy bodies caregivers.
Where: Nassau County; call for location.
Address: Nassau County; call for location. Lynbook, NY 11563
Who to Contact:
Norma Loeb
212.556.1278
normalanne@gmail.com

New York Metro Area Support Group
Meeting Dates and Times: Second Tuesday of every month, 12:30 p.m. – 2:00 p.m.
Who: LBD caregivers.
Where: Manhattan; call for location.

Address: Manhattan; call for location. Manhattan; call for location., NY 10018
Who to Contact:
Norma Loeb
212.556.1278
normalanne@gmail.com

Mid-Ohio Dementia–Related Diseases (LBD, Alzheimer's Disease, PDD) Education and Support Group
Meeting Dates and Times: Third Tuesday of every month, 7:00 p.m. – 8:30 p.m.
Who: Family, friends and care providers of loved ones with dementia-related diseases.
Where: Our Saviors Lutheran Church
Address: 725 East Eliza Street Kenton, OH 43326
Who to Contact:
Melody Hampton
937.354.3322 or 419.674.7345
hampt0ns@embarqmail.com

Northwest Ohio Dementia-Related Diseases (LBD, PDD, Alzheimer's Disease) Support Group
Meeting Dates and Times: Third Thursday of every month, 7:00 p.m. – 8:30 p.m.
Who: Caregivers, family, and friends of those with dementia-related diseases.
Where: Hilty Memorial Home, Conference Room
Address: 304 Hilty Drive Pandora, OH 45877
Who to Contact:
Ruth Ann Grismore
419.634.2282
frgrismore@embarqmail.com

Edmond Santa Fe Dementia Caregivers Support Group
Meeting Dates and Times: Second Monday of every month, 7:00 p.m. – 8:30 p.m.

Who: For caregivers and family members of those diagnosed with Dementia with Lewy bodies, Alzheimer's Disease and other types of dementia.
Where: Santa Fe Presbyterian Church
Address: 1603 North Santa Fe Edmond, OK 73003
Who to Contact:
Cindy Thomas
405.715.9954
Cynthia-thomas@ouhsc.edu

Alzheimer Society of Toronto Lewy Body Family Support Group
Meeting Dates and Times: Second Wednesday of every month 4:30 p.m. – 6:00 p.m.
Who: Family members of those diagnosed with Dementia with Lewy bodies.
Where: Alzheimer Society of Toronto
Address: 20 Eglinton Avenue West, 16th Floor Toronto, ON M4R 1K8
Who to Contact:
Christine Leskovar
416.322.6560, ext.6304
cleskovar@alzheimertoronto.org

Kingston Dementia with Lewy bodies Support Group
Meeting Dates and Times: Second Thursday of every month, 7 p.m. - 9 p.m.
Who: For caregivers of people with Dementia with Lewy bodies.
Where: The Royal George
Address: 5 Gore Street Kingston, ON K7L0A1
Who to Contact:
Peggy Brown
613.766.1943
maggystillyoung@yahoo.ca

Bucks County Dementia with Lewy bodies Support Group
Meeting Dates and Times: Third Tuesday of every month, 2 p.m. – 4 p.m.
Who: For caregivers, family members, and friends experiencing the daily struggles of LBD.
Where: The Manor at York Town
Address: 2010 York Road Jamison, PA 18929
Who to Contact:
Cammy Frazier
215.766.8929
camcat65@verizon.net
Home Instead Senior Care Plumsteadville
215.766.1617

Susquehanna Valley Dementia with Lewy bodies Support Group
Meeting Dates and Times: First Tuesday of every month, 7:00 p.m. - 9:00 p.m.
Who: For caregivers, family members, and friends experiencing the daily struggles of LBD.
Where: St Peter's Lutheran Church
Address: 10 Delp Road Lancaster, PA 17601
Who to Contact:
Kim Lemon MacIver
717.572.9908
kim.kitten.lemon@gmail.com
Sandy Smith
717.285.2579
meadowview@embarqmail.com
St Peter's Lutheran Church
717.569.9211

Beaufort County Dementia Support Group
Meeting Dates and Times: Second Monday of each month, 10:00 am-11:00am

Who: Caregivers and family members of those diagnosed with Dementia with Lewy bodiess and related dementias.
Where: Riverside at Belfair
Address: 60 Oak Forest Road Bluffton, SC 29910
Who to Contact:
Dianne Hillyear
843.290.6560
Dianne@riversideatbelfair.com

East Cooper Dementia Caregiver Education and Support Group

Meeting Dates and Times: First and third Wednesday of every month, 9:30 a.m. – 10:30 a.m.
Who: Caregivers, family members, friends, and health care professionals in the greater Charleston/tri-county area caring for persons with progressive forms of dementia from diseases such as Dementia with Lewy bodies, Alzheimer's disease, Pick's disease, vascular dementia, frontotemperal dementia, or Parkinson's disease.
Where: All Saints Lutheran Church
Address: 2107 Highway 17 North Mt. Pleasant, SC 29464
Who to Contact:
Ginger Deignan
843.810.5576
respitecare@comcast.net

Upstate Dementia with Lewy bodies Support Group

Meeting Dates and Times: First Tuesday of every month, 5:00 p.m. – 6:00 p.m.
Who: Caregivers, family members, friends, support persons and health care professionals, in Greenville, Greer, Easley, and Spartanburg, caring for persons with Dementia with Lewy bodies, Alzheimer's disease, and other types of degenerative dementias.
Where: The Haven in the Village at Chanticleer
Address: 355 Berkmans Lane Greenville, SC 29605
Who to Contact:

Gail Stokes
864.350.7160
gstokes@SeniorLivingNow.com

Nashville and Bellevue Lewy Body and Other Dementias Support Group
Meeting Dates and Times: Second Tuesday of every other month, 1:00 p.m.-2:30 p.m.
Who: For caregivers and family members who have a loved one with Dementia with Lewy bodies, Alzheimer's disease, or any other dementia.
Where: Bellevue Family YMCA's J.L. Turner Center
Address: 8101 Highway 100 Nashville, TN 37221
Who to Contact:
Marshall Snyder
615.403.5067
marshall.snyder1@gmail.com

Austin Dementia with Lewy bodies Support Group Meeting
Meeting Dates and Times: Last Saturday of every month, 9:30 a.m. – 11:00 a.m.
Who: LBD caregivers, family and friends
Where: Austin Groups for the Elderly
Address: 3710 Cedar St. Austin, TX 78705
Who to Contact:
Kelli Cotner
512.904.9101

Houston Area Dementia with Lewy bodies and Parkinson's Caregivers Support Group
Meeting Dates and Times: Fourth Monday of every month, 10:30 a.m. – 12 p.m.
Who: For caregivers and family members of those diagnosed with LBD and Parkinson's disease.
Where: Red Cross of Greater Houston
Address: 2700 SW Freeway Houston, TX 77030

Who to Contact:
Michelle Sonnier
713.314.1393
michelle.sonnier@alz.org

Houston Area Men's Caregivers Support Group
Meeting Dates and Times: First Tuesday of every month, 1:30 p.m. – 3:00 p.m.
Who: Male caregivers caring for a spouse with any type of dementia.
Where: Alzheimer's Association
Address: 2242 W. Holcombe Blvd Houston, TX 77030
Who to Contact:
Michelle Sonnier
713.314.1393
michelle.sonnier@alz.org

Houston Area Support Group
Meeting Dates and Times: Third Saturday of every month (except for July (no meeting) and December, when the meeting is on the second Saturday.) 1:00 p.m. – 3:00 p.m.
Who: For caregivers and persons with progressive supranuclear palsy (PSP), Dementia with Lewy bodies, corticobasal ganglionic degeneration, and multiple system atrophy.
Where: Memorial Hermann Southwest Hospital, Professional Building II, Learning Center B
Address: 7737 Beechnut Street Houston, TX 77074
Who to Contact:
Karen M. Kennemer
281.358.2282
kmk1224@aol.com

North Dallas/Richardson Dementia with Lewy bodies Caregivers Support Group
Meeting Dates and Times: First Wednesday of every month, 5:00 p.m. – 6:00 p.m.

Who: For caregivers and family members of those diagnosed with LBD.
Where: Friends Place Adult Day Services
Address: 1960 Nantucket Drive Richardson, TX 75080
Who to Contact:
Pam Kovacs
972.437.2940
pamkovacs@friendsplaceads.com

Salt Lake Valley LBD Support Group
Meeting Dates and Times: Who to Contact Raquel Asay for details.
Who: For caregivers and family members of those diagnosed with Lewy body disease.
Where: Who to Contact Raquel Asay for details.
Address: Who to Contact Raquel Asay for details. Who to Contact Raquel Asay for details., UT 99999
Who to Contact:
Raquel Asay
801.533.0972
rachelar39@gmail.com

Central Virginia Lewy Body and Other Dementias Support Group
Meeting Dates and Times: Fourth Thursday of every month, 3 p.m. – 4 p.m.
Who: Caregivers and family members of those diagnosed with dementia-related diseases, such as LBD, PDD, Alzheimer's disease.
Where: Lynchburg Family Medicine Conference Room
Address: 2323 Memorial Ave., Suite 10 Lynchburg, VA 24501
Who to Contact:
Jean Driscoll
540.580.9000
jdrisc@live.com

Northern Vermont Early Onset Dementia Support Group

Meeting Dates and Times: Meeting Dates and Times: Second Tuesday of every month, 5:30 p.m. – 7 p.m.
Who: For people under 65 with a diagnosis of dementia and their spouse or partner.
Where: The Arbors
Address: 687 Harbor Road Shelburne, VT 05482
Who to Contact:
Rachel Cummings
802.288.8117
armisteadcare@comcast.net
Kathi Monteith
802.985.8600
kmonteith@benchmarkquality.com

Central Washington Dementia with Lewy bodies, Alzheimer's Disease and Other Dementias Support Group

Meeting Dates and Times: Fourth Tuesday of every month, 6:30 p.m. - 8:00 p.m. Begins February 22, 2011.
Who: For caregivers and family members who have a loved one with Dementia with Lewy bodies, Alzheimer's Disease or any other related dementia
Where: Orchard House Assisted Living and Memory Care
Address: 2001 West 5th Street Grandview, WA 98930
Who to Contact:
Gaylene Tucker
509.391.0306
gaylene_cci@clearwire.net
Jana Bell
509.308.5667
cwdementiagroup@clearwire.net

Central Washington Dementia with Lewy bodies, Alzheimer's Disease and Other Dementias Support Group

Meeting Dates and Times: Fourth Tuesday of every month, 6:30 p.m. - 8:00 p.m. Begins February 22, 2011.
Who: For caregivers and family members who have a loved one with Dementia with Lewy bodies, Alzheimer's Disease or any other related dementia.
Where: Orchard House, Assisted Living and Memory Care
Address: 2001 West 5th Street Grandview, WA 98930
Who to Contact:
Gaylene Tucker
509.391.0306
gaylene_cci@clearwire.net
Jana Bell
509.308.5667
cwdementiagroup@clearwire.net

Chippewa Valley LBD Caregiver Support Group
Meeting Dates and Times: Second Wednesday of every month, 6 p.m. - 8 p.m.
Who: For caregivers and family members of a loved one with Dementia with Lewy bodies.
Where: Sacred Heart Hospital
Address: 900 West Clairemont Avenue - Conference Room #15 Eau Claire, WI 54701
Who to Contact:
Amy Lokken
715.379.3148
amy@modularmarketingsystems.com

Columbus Dementia Caregiver Support Group
Meeting Dates and Times: Second Tuesday of every month, 10:00 a.m. – 11:30 a.m.
Who: Caregivers and family members who have a loved one with Dementia with Lewy bodies or any other dementia.
Where: Columbus Community Hospital, Emerald Room
Address: 1515 Park Avenue Columbus, WI 53925
Who to Contact:

Carol Olson
608.742.9055
carol.olson@alzwisc.org
Carol Olson
608.963.2688
carol.olson@alzwisc.org

Reedsburg Dementia Caregiver Support Group
Meeting Dates and Times: Third Wednesday of every month, noon – 1:30 p.m.
Who: Caregivers and family members who have a loved one with Dementia with Lewy bodies or any other dementia.
Where: Reedsburg Area Senior Life Center
Address: 2350 N. Dewey Ave. Reedsburg, WI 53939
Who to Contact:
Carol Olson
608.742.9055
carol.olson@alzwisc.org
Carol Olson
608.963.2688
carol.olson@alzwisc.org

Southern Wisconsin/Beloit (daytime) Dementia Support Group
Meeting Dates and Times: Second and fourth Tuesday of every month, 1:00 p.m. – 2:30 p.m.
Who: Caregivers of individuals with Dementia with Lewy bodies, Alzheimer's disease, and other related illnesses.
Where: Beloit Memorial Hospital
Address: 1969 West Hart Road Beloit, WI 53511
Who to Contact:
Larisa Chmielewski
608.314.8500

Southern Wisconsin/Beloit (evening) Dementia Support Group

Meeting Dates and Times: Third Tuesday of every month, 7:00 p.m. – 8:30 p.m.
Who: Caregivers of individuals with Dementia with Lewy bodies, Alzheimer's disease, and other related illnesses.
Where: First Methodist Church
Address: 511 Public Avenue Beloit, WI 53511
Who to Contact:
Nancy Toubl
608.362.8866
Julie Ojeda
608.365.5529

Southern Wisconsin/Edgerton Dementia Support Group
Meeting Dates and Times: Third Wednesday of every month, 1:00 p.m. – 2:30 p.m.
Who: Caregivers of individuals with Dementia with Lewy bodies, Alzheimer's disease, and other related illnesses.
Where: Edgerton Hospital (in the classroom near the cafeteria on the outpatient floor)
Address: 313 Stoughton Road Edgerton, WI 53534
Who to Contact:
Tammy Pence
608.314.8500

Southern Wisconsin/Janesville Dementia Support Group
Meeting Dates and Times: Second Thursday of every month, 10:00 a.m. – 11:30 a.m.
Who: Caregivers of individuals with Dementia with Lewy bodies, Alzheimer's disease, and other related illnesses.
Where: American Red Cross
Address: 211 North Parker Drive Janesville, WI 53545
Who to Contact:
Julie Seeman
608.758.8455
Paulette Steinke
608.758.8455

KYOWVA (Kentucky, Ohio and West Virginia) Lewy Body and Other Dementias Support Group
Meeting Dates and Times: First Thursday of every month, 6:30 p.m. – 8:30 p.m.
Who: Dementia caregivers, including Dementia with Lewy bodies caregivers.
Where: Sarah Care
Address: 2 Courtyard Lane Barboursville, WV 25504
Who to Contact:
Kelly Shivel
304.736.3005
kwshivel@aol.com

LBD Glossary

Acetylcholine – a major neurotransmitter released by brain cells (neurons) and is essential in carrying information between brain cells. It is involved in sensation, cognition, emotion and arousal. Loss of acetylcholine-producing neurons may lead to Alzheimer's disease and Lewy body dementia.

Acetylcholinesterase inhibitor (achei) – also called cholinesterase inhibitor or anticholinesterase, these drugs work by inhibiting the breakdown of acetylcholine thus increasing its levels in the brain – at the same time, cognitive symptoms of dementia are decreased,

Action tremor -- refer to a tremor that is present when the limbs and trunk are actively maintained in certain positions and may persist throughout active movement.

Activities of daily living (ADL) -- daily activities such as eating, grooming, bathing and toileting. Tasks, which, patients with movement disorders like dementia may have difficulty performing alone

Adult daycare -- a non-residential facility where adults have the opportunity to interact with others, socialize and at the same time, undergo physical therapy. Staff includes nurses, nursing assistants, physical therapists and occupational therapists

Advance directives – divided into three categories: living will, power of attorney and health care proxy, these are legal documents concerning a patient's treatment preference. In an event that the patient can no longer make medical decisions on his/her own behalf, a surrogate decision maker is designated.

Adverse drug reactions -- unintended and undesired effects of medications that occur at a dosage intended for prevention and treatment.

Agitation – also referred to as psychomotor agitation, this involves excessive behavioral or motor activity such as pacing and jittery movements often associated with restlessness and anxiety.

Agitated depression – Persistent restlessness and agitation in Major depressive disorder

Agnosia – inability to recognize sound, smell or objects despite intact senses.

Akathisia – a subjective feeling of restlessness manifested a compelling need to be in constant movement; be seen as an extrapyramidal adverse effect of antipsychotic medication

Akinesia -- Lack of physical movement as in the extreme immobility seen in catatonic patients

Alpha-synuclein -- a protein prominently expressed in the central nervous system, aggregates of which form the essential component of Lewy bodies

Alzheimer's disease – a neurodegenerative disease affecting the brain characterized by language and memory impairment, disorientation to time, place and person and personality changes

Ambulatory – ability to walk and move about without assistance

Ambulatory care – service given to patients seen on an outpatient basis which includes a thorough history making and physical examination, diagnosis, treatment and rehabilitation

Amnesia – Partial or total inability to recall past experiences

Amyloid – aggregates of proteins deposited in tissues

Anhidrosis -- Partial or total inability to sweat seen in diabetes, Parkinson's disease and Lewy body dementias as a result of nerve damage

Anosmia – refers to the inability to smell and can either be transitional or permanent.

Anticholinergic – drugs used to counter the effect of acetylcholine in the body; these are particularly utilized in reducing muscle cramps and spasms

Anticholinesterase: See acetylcholinesterase inhibitor.

Antidepressants – drugs used to treat depression, which includes monoamine inhibitors, serotonin selective reuptake inhibitors and Tricyclics.

Antipsychotic drug – also known as neuroleptics, these are drugs used to treat symptoms of Schizophrenia (eg. Hallucinations, delusions, agitations).

Anxiety -- Feeling of apprehension caused by anticipation of danger often manifested with profuse sweating, rapid heart rate and muscle tension.

Anxiolytic: Drugs used to treat the symptoms of anxiety.

Apathy – partial or total lack of emotion and social withdrawal

Aphasia – manifested as either the inability to express and/or understand verbal language brought about by a damage to the brain

Apraxia -- a state in which an attentive patient loses the ability to execute previously learned activities in the absence of weakness, sensory loss, or extrapyramidal derangement that would be adequate to explain the deficit.

Apraxia of speech – a speech disorder in which a person has trouble saying what he or she wants to say correctly and consistently.

Assisted living facility – a long term care facility which may be part of a retirement community or nursing home, designed for disabled persons and elderlies who may require assistance in carrying out activities of daily living but do not necessarily need a full-time nursing care

Ataxia – lack of coordination and unsteadiness seen in persons with neurologic disorders

Atrophy – reduction in size of an organ or tissue resulting from a decrease in cell size and number. It is also referred to as wasting

Attention deficit -- diminished ability to sustain attention

Atypical antipsychotic drug – these refers to the newer generation antipsychotic medications with lesser or no extrapyramidal symptoms compared to typical antipsychotic drugs.

Auditory hallucination: False perception of sound, usually voices, but also other noises, such as music.

Aura -- Warning sensations, such as automatisms, fullness in the stomach, blushing, and visual disturbances, such as the perception of lights usually experienced before a seizure or migraine headache

Autonomic nervous system – a division of the Peripheral nervous system that involves mainly in the regulation of body processes such as digestion, salivation, heart rate and perspiration. It is further divided into the sympathetic nervous system and the parasympathetic nervous system.

Basal ganglia – area in the brain responsible for motor control, learning and cognition. This is affected in conditions such as Huntington's disease and Parkinson's

Benzodiazepine – a psychoactive drug used to treat panic attacks, anxiety, insomnia or seizure

Binswanger disease -- also known as subcortical vascular dementia and subcortical leukoencephalopathy, this refers to a rare form of dementia characterized by the presence of many small infarctions of the white matter that spare the cortical regions

Biomarker – a substance found in tissues or body fluids used to detect the presence of a disease or measure its severity

Black box warning – a notice seen in prescription packages of medications that indicates any significant serious or life-threatening adverse effects. This is issued by the Food and Drug Administration to assure consumer safety.

Bradykinesia – connotes a slowness of movement characterized by a prolonged time of execution

Brain stem – posterior part of the brain that connects the cerebrum and spinal cord. It functions for the regulation of breathing, sleep cycle and heart rate

Capgras syndrome – a delusion of misidentification which refers to the belief that a familiar person has been replaced by an impostor

Case management – a coordinated plan of action performed by health care professionals in the management of a particular illness

Central nervous system (CNS) – a division of the nervous system consisting of the brain and spinal cord

Cerebellum – a part of the brain involved in coordination of movements and balance

Cerebral – a term used in reference to the brain or the cerebrum, in particular

Cerebral cortex – the outer covering of the cerebrum also known as the gray matter

Cerebrospinal fluid (CSF) – clear, bodily fluid that surrounds and acts as a cushion preventing injury in the brain and spinal cord

Cerebrovascular – a term used in reference to the blood vessels that supply the brain

Cerebrovascular disease: any abnormality of the brain resulting from a pathologic process of the blood vessels supplying it

Cerebrum – The largest part of the brain located above the cerebellum and brainstem and is divided into the right and left hemispheres

Cholinesterase – enzyme that breaks down acetylcholine

Cholinesterase inhibitor: See acetylcholinesterase.

Clinical psychologist – a non-MD professional that specializes in the diagnosis and management of brain diseases, emotional and behavioral problems through methods such as talk therapy or cognitive behavioral therapy

Clinical psychology: -- a field of psychology that s concerned with the diagnosis, treatment and prevention of mental illnesses

Clinical trials – research studies conducted to human subjects which aims to evaluate the efficacy and safety of a certain medication or medical devices

Cognition-- a mental process which encompasses the aspects of awareness, memory, judgment and reasoning

Cognitive – pertains to cognition

Computerized Axial Tomography (CAT or CT) – a diagnostic tool that utilizes x-ray images to generate cross-sectional views of body organs and tissues with the aid of a computer

Competency – ability of an individual to participate in legal proceedings

COMT inhibitors -- drugs that inhibit the action of the enzyme Catechol-O-methyl transferase
(COMT)

Confabulation – refers to the unconscious making up of false answers when memory is impaired. This may involve imagining experiences or events that have no basis in fact

Conservator – a person appointed by the court to oversee the financial and personal affairs of those proven to have physical or mental limitations and are unable to do so

Convalescent home: See nursing home.

Cortex – refers to the outer layer of the cerebellum and cerebrum

Creutzfeldt-Jakob disease – a rapidly progressive disorder caused by a transmissible infectious protein known as a prion that affects the cerebral cortex and basal ganglia. It is characterized by a rapidly progressive dementia and gradual loss of muscle control

Deep brain stimulation (DBS) -- a surgical procedure that involves implantation of brain pacemakers in an aim to treat disorders such as Parkinson's disease

Delusion: a false belief, based on incorrect inference about external reality, that is held firmly despite objective and obvious contradictory proof or evidence and despite the fact that other members of the culture do not share the belief

Delusional misidentification syndrome – a delusional disorder characterized by a false belief that a person, place or object has been modified or replaced
-- see Capgras syndrome

Dementia: Mental disorder characterized by general impairment in intellectual functioning without clouding of consciousness; characterized by failing memory, difficulty with calculations, distractibility, alterations in mood and affect, impaired judgment and abstraction, reduced facility with language, and disturbance of orientation

Dementia–capable -- health professional skilled in working with patients with dementia

Dementia with Lewy bodies (DLB): See Lewy body dementias.

Depressant: -- medications that reduces the activity of the central nervous system hence, depressing arousal levels manifested as sleepiness, muscle relaxation and slowed breathing

Depression -- Mental state characterized by feelings of sadness, loneliness, despair, low self-esteem, and self-reproach; accompanying signs include psychomotor retardation or, at times, agitation, withdrawal from interpersonal contact, and vegetative symptoms, such as insomnia and anorexia

Disinhibition: refers to the freedom to act in accordance with inner drives or feelings and with less regard for restraints dictated by cultural norms or one's superego.

Dizziness: a general term used to describe feelings of lightheadedness, faintness and vertigo with/without associated disturbances in vision

Dopamine – a neurotransmitter that plays an important role in cognition, motivation and pleasure. Loss of dopamine-producing neurons results in the motor symptoms of Parkinson's disease

Dopamine agonist: medications used to treat Parkinson's disease which works by mimicking the action of dopamine resulting to the activation of dopamine receptors

Drug induced parkinsonism – Parkinson-like symptoms, usually reversible, caused as a side effect of some medications

Durable power of attorney – a legal document which enables another person to act on another person's behalf in cases of an incapacitating medical condition

Dysarthria: slurred speech because of incoordination of speech muscles

Dysautonomia: malfunctioning of the autonomic nervous system

Dyskinesia Difficulty in performing movements which may occur as a side effect of antipsychotic medications

Dysphagia: Difficulty in swallowing defined as a sensation of "sticking" or obstruction of the passage of food through the mouth, pharynx, or esophagus

Dysphasia Difficulty in comprehending oral language (reception dysphasia) or in trying to express verbal language (expressive dysphasia)

Dysphonia -- Difficulty or pain in speaking.

Dysphoria: Feeling of unpleasantness or discomfort; a mood of general dissatisfaction and restlessness that occurs in depression and anxiety

Dyspnea – difficulty in breathing

Dysthymia: -- a chronic form of depression less severe than major depression and usually lasts less than 2 years

Dystonia: Extrapyramidal motor disturbance consisting of slow, sustained contractions of the axial or appendicular musculature; one movement often predominates, leading to relatively sustained postural deviations

Early-onset familial Alzheimer's disease -- Alzheimer's disease that occurs before the age of 65

End stage: the last stage of a progressive terminal disease

Elder law attorney – a lawyer that specializes and practices in the area of law that focuses on issues that affects older adults

Essential tremor: a condition wherein a person shakes or trembles uncontrollably during voluntary movement

Euphoria: Exaggerated feeling of well-being that is inappropriate to real events that can occur with drugs such as opiates, amphetamines, and alcohol

Excessive daytime somnolence (EDS – refers to the tendency to fall asleep intermittently during the day despite sufficient sleep at night

Executive dysfunction – disruption of the executive brain functions which includes problem solving, attention, organization and decision making

Explicit memory: memory that needs conscious recollection for it to be recalled; this typically declines with age and is affected with dementia

Facial affect -- emotion displayed to others through facial expression

Familial -- tendency of a disease to occur among family members that is not attributed to chance alone

Festinating gait: type of gait characterized by short, rapid steps with associated shuffling and rigidity

Fluctuating cognition: a symptom of dementia characterized by the waxing and waning of thinking skills, speech ability and alertness

Flushing – an involuntary response manifested as reddening of the face and neck

Foley catheter: -- a flexible plastic tube inserted into the bladder for continuous drainage of urine

Frontal lobe – front area of the brain responsible for functions such as planning, organizing, problem solving, selective attention, emotion, personality and social behavior

Frontotemporal dementia: -- a type of dementia that affects primarily the frontal and temporal lobes of the brain

Gait – a manner of moving on foot

Geriatric care worker – A professional which specializes in the care of the elderly

Geriatric psychiatrist – a psychiatrist who specializes in the diagnosis and management of mental and behavioral disorders affecting the elderly

Geriatric medicine -- a branch of medicine that specializes in the diagnosis, management and prevention of diseases affecting the elderly

Geriatrician – a physician specializing in geriatric medicine; working directly with elderly patients

Gerontologist – a professional specializing in gerontology, the study of aging

Gerontology – a comprehensive study of the aging process and the problems of the aged

Glutamate: -- primary excitatory neurotransmitter

Guardian – a person appointed by court and authorized to make legal and financial decisions on another person's behalf

Gustatory hallucination – false perception primary involving the sense of taste

Hallucination -- False sensory perception occurring in the absence of any relevant external stimulation of the sensory modality involved

Healthcare proxy: a legal document that grants a power of attorney to an individual allowing him/her to make medical decisions on another person's behalf in case of incapacitation

Hereditary – transmitted from parent to offspring

Home health agency: organization that specializes in the provision of in-home health care services

Home health care – refers to the provision of in-home health care services such as nursing care and physical therapy

Hospice – a facility that aims to provide end-of-life care to persons with terminal illnesses

Hospice care – supportive care given to patients with terminal illnesses which focuses on improved quality of life and general comfort rather than cure

Huntington's disease -- a neurodegenerative genetic disorder characterized by jerky, uncontrolled movements and cognitive impairments

Hypnagogic hallucination Hallucination occurring while falling asleep

Hypnopompic hallucination -- Hallucination occurring while awakening from sleep

Hypokinesia: an abnormal decrease in motor activity

Hypophonia – an abnormally weak voice resulting from incoordination of the vocal muscles

Idiopathic: any disease of unknown cause

Illusions: Perceptual misinterpretation of a real external stimulus

Implicit memory: a type of long-term memory that is automatic and allows a person to learn things without conscious thought

Incontinence: loss of bladder (Urinary incontinence) or bowel (Fecal incontinence) control

Insomnia: Difficulty in falling asleep or difficulty in staying asleep

Intention tremor: tremor that occurs when a person aims for a target (as when reaching for an object with the hand).

Instrumental activities of daily living (iadls): activities such as writing or using the telephone which are not necessary for basic functioning but required for independent living

Irritability: excessive emotional response often associated with anger and frustration

Kinesthetic hallucination – false perception of bodily movement

Late onset Alzheimer's disease: Alzheimer's disease that occurs after 65 years old

Lewy bodies – abnormal protein aggregates comprised primarily of alpha-synuclein seen in patients with Parkinson's disease

Lewy body dementias (LBD): a progressive, degenerative form of dementia characterized by loss of spontaneous movement, rigidity, tremor, shuffling gait, cognitive and behavioral changes. Its is associated with the deposition of Lewy bodies in certain areas of the brain

Licensed clinical professional counselor (LCPC) – health professionals trained in psychotherapy

Lilliputian hallucination: Visual sensation that persons or objects are reduced in size

Living will: an advance directive wherein a person directs treatment preferences in end-of-life situations.

Long term care (LTC): care given to patients with chronic disability or illnesses given either at home or at a medical facility

Long term care facility (LTCF): facility that offers long term care to patients with chronic disability or illnesses

Long term memory (LTM): system in which information is stored and managed permanently for long term use

Major depression – a condition characterized by the persistence of a depressed mood often associated with suicidal thoughts, weight loss, feelings of hopelessness and insomnia

Magnetic resonance imaging (MRI) – a diagnostic tool that utilizes a magnetic field in order to produce images of internal body structures

Managed care – a program in health care delivery that minimizes costs without compromising healthcare quality

MAO inhibitor – medications used to treat depression that acts by inhibiting monoamine oxidase thereby reducing dopamine breakdown

Mask-like face – a complete lack of facial expression or affect

Medicaid: A healthcare program which aims to provide quality healthcare benefits to persons with insufficient income and resources in the United States

Medicare (Canada): universal health care program in Canada funded by the public

Medicare (United States): health insurance program that targets those aged 65 and older or those with conditions such as kidney failure

Medicare Part A (United States): Medicare program covering for inpatient hospital stays

Medicare Part B (United States): Medicare program covering for outpatient services

Medicare Part C (United States): an option given to those in Medicare Part A or B to have their health benefits received through a private insurance plan

Medicare Part D (United States -- Medicare program for anyone enrolled in Part A or B that covers prescription medications

Medication management: process of monitoring medications a patient takes in order to confirm that the patient is complying with a medication regimen

Medigap (United States): Private health insurance plans intended to supplement Medicare
Benefits and hence, fill the gaps in healthcare coverage.

Memory: Process by which past events and knowledge are stored and recalled. It is damaged in disorders such as dementia

Memory span: the number of items that a person can recall

Mini Mental State Examination (MMSE): A brief exam often used to screen for dementia, conducted to determine a person's level of basic cognitive skills such as memory, language use, attention and comprehension.

Mood stabilizer: Drugs used to treat mania and agitation in bipolar disorder15

Multiple system atrophy (MSA): a Degenerative disorder characterized by incontinence, dry mouth, slurred speech and loss of muscle coordination resulting from damage to the autonomic nervous system

Musical hallucination: false perception of music

National Institutes of Health (NIH): United States government health agency devoted to medical research

National Institute of Mental Health (NIMH): A component organization of the National Institutes of Health which conducts and funds researches pertaining to mental health in the bid to better understand, prevent and treat psychiatric conditions

National Institute of Neurological Disorders and Stroke (NINDS): A component organization
Of the National Institutes of Health which conducts and supports researches on the causes, diagnosis and treatment of neurological diseases in an aim to lessen the burden of neurological diseases

National Institute on Aging (NIA): A component organization of the National Institutes of Health which supports and conducts researches regarding aging and age related diseases in an aim to better understand the aging process.

Nerve: cordlike bundle of fibers in the peripheral nervous system that functions in the transmission of sensory and motor signals in the body

Nerve cell: See neuron.

Nervous system: a complex organ system composed of the brain, spinal cord and its corresponding network of nerve fibers responsible for the coordination of body processes

Neurofibrillary tangles: aggregates of paired helical filaments composed primarily of abnormally formed tau protein found in the nerve cells of those with Alzheimer's disease

Neurodegenerative: progressive loss of function and degeneration of neurons

Neuroleptic: refers to antipsychotic medications

Neuroleptic drugs/neuroleptics: See antipsychotic drug.

Neuroleptic malignant syndrome (NMS): Manifested as high fever, muscular rigidity, unstable blood pressure and autonomic dysfunction, this is a rare neurologic disorder caused by adverse reaction to neuroleptic drugs

Neuroleptic sensitivity: a collection of Parkinson-like manifestations such as rigidity and gait problems resulting from intake of neuroleptic drugs

Neurological: pertains to the nervous system

Neurologist: Physician who specializes in the diagnosis and treatment of diseases of the nervous system

Neurology: a branch of medicine that deals with the diagnosis and treatment of diseases involving the nervous system

Neuron: nerve cells that serves as the building block of the nervous system. It process and transmit information via electrical and chemical signals from one part of the body to another.

Neuropathologist: Pathologist who specializes in diseases of the nervous system and arrives at the diagnosis through direct tissue examination by performing a biopsy or autopsy

Neuropathy: a collection of disorders involving the nerves of the peripheral nervous system

Neuropsychiatrist: a physician who specializes in both psychiatry and neurology

Neuropsychologist: Psychologist who specializes in brain disorders and has completed the required special training

Neuropsychological test: specifically designed tasks used to measure cognitive function. Location and extent of brain injury is determined by the degree of impairment of a particular skill

Neurotransmitter – chemicals released by neurons which functions in signal transmission leading in either an increase or decrease in the activity of the receiving neuron

NMDA antagonist: medications used mainly as anesthetics which acts by inhibiting the action of N-methyl d-aspartate (NMDA).

Nurse, licensed practical (LPN): nurses who has earned a state or national license after completing the training program for nursing

Nurse, licensed vocational (LVN): refers to licensed practical nurse in California and Texas

Nurse practitioner (NP): -- registered nurses who ha completed a master's degree or an advanced training program

Nurse, registered (RN): refers to those who has accomplished all requirements in the nursing program (ie. Completion of a 2-4 year course in nursing and provision of direct patient care in a clinical setting)

Nursing home – residential care facility designed for patients with chronic illnesses particularly the elderlies who may need continuous support in carrying out activities of daily living

Nursing assistant (CAN) – a person who has undergone and completed a health care training program and has provided routine patient care

Occupational therapist (OT) – professionals working with persons with temporary or permanent disability in an aim to develop, improve, sustain or restore the highest possible level of independence

Olfactory hallucination: false perception involving the sense of smell

Ombudsman: a person who investigates complaints made by the public against an institution or corporation

Orthostatic hypotension – decrease in blood pressure upon standing resulting in a momentary reduction in blood flow to the brain manifested by fainting, blurring of vision or dizziness

Palilalia: repetition of a word or syllable

Palliative care: care intended to alleviate disease symptoms and to ensure improvement in the quality of life of patients. It is not designed to change the course of the disease or to provide cure.

Parasympathetic nervous system (PNS): a division of the autonomic nervous system which when activated results in the decrease of heart rate, stimulation of digestion, papillary constriction and relaxation of sphincter muscles

Parkinson's disease (PD): a neurologic disorder characterized by postural instability, resting tremors and rigidity, attributed to the loss of dopamine-producing neurons

Parkinson's disease dementia (PDD): See Lewy body dementias.

Parkinsonism: refers to symptoms that resemble that of Parkinson's disease

Parkinsonian – refers to the symptoms of Parkinsonism or Parkinson's disease

Peripheral nervous system – a network of nerves and ganglia outside the brain and spinal cord

Pharm.D (Doctor of Pharmacy): Professional degree required to become a registered pharmacist.

Physical therapy (PT): a branch of rehabilitative medicine that aims to maintain and improve functional movement by employing special exercises to patients

Physician assistant (PA): a Health professional working under the supervision of a licensed physician and has completed a 2 year physician assistant program

Pick's disease: a form of dementia characterized by a preponderance of atrophy in the frontotemporal regions and abnormal deposits called Pick bodies inside the neurons

Plaques – typically seen in Alzheimer's disease, these are abnormal protein deposits embedded in abnormally distended neurons

Positron emission tomography (PET): a diagnostic tool that utilizes radioactive tracers injected in the body allowing physicians to view the body's metabolic activity

Postural instability: inability to maintain correct standing or sitting posture

Power of attorney: a written authorization that allows a person to act on someone else's behalf in a legal or business matter

Progressive: advancement of the disease entity or an increase in severity

Progressive supranuclear palsy (PSP): a rapidly progressing degenerative disease with patients manifesting problems in motor and eye movement

Propulsive gait: See festinating gait.

Protein -- molecules composed of amino acid chains forming essential nutrients in the body

Psychiatrist: a physician who specializes in the diagnosis and treatment of mental disorders.

Psychologist: a professional who studies human behavior and mental processes

Psychomotor: term used with reference to cognition and its associated motor activity

Psychopharmacology – deals with the study of medications used to treat psychiatric disorders

Psychosis: Mental disorder in which the thoughts, affective response, ability to recognize reality, and ability to communicate and relate to others are sufficiently impaired to interfere grossly with the capacity to deal with reality

Psychosocial – pertaining to both psychological and social aspects of human behavior

Rapid eye movement sleep (REM): stage of sleep characterized by rapid eye movements and the predominance of dreams. Rapid, low voltage theta waves are seen in EEG tracing during this state. Also, metabolism and blood flow are restored to the levels of the waking state during REM sleep.

Receptor – structures located in the cell surface which receive signals from outside of the cell

REM sleep behavior disorder (RBD) -- occurring exclusively during REM sleep, an individual tends to act out their dreams often violently resulting in injury to self and bedmates. An early manifestation of a degenerative brain disease, this result from the disruption of the normal sleep paralysis preventing muscle relaxation during REM sleep

Resting tremor: tremors that occurs at rest and stops with voluntary movement

Retropulsion: a tendency to fall backwards seen in patients with gait disorders resulting from a sudden loss of balance

Rigidity: resistance to passive movement due to increased muscle tone

Safe Return: a nationwide program that assists in the identification and safe return of persons with Alzheimer's and other related disorders who wander and become lost

Sedative: See depressant.

21

Short term memory: responsible for the momentary processing and storage of recent memories

Skilled nursing facility (SNF): an institution which aims to provide daily medical care, rehabilitation and general assistance to the elderly and persons with disabilities

Sleep apnea: momentary cessation of breathing which occurs during sleep which can lead to poor sleep quality and excessive sleepiness during the day

SNRI (Serotonin-norepinephrine reuptake inhibitor): medications used to treat depression, anxiety and obsessive-compulsive disorders which acts by increasing serotonin and norepinephrine levels in the brain

Somatic hallucination: See tactile hallucination.

Somnolent: Sleepy or drowsy. See also excessive daytime somnolence.

Spasmodic dysphonia: a voice disorder resulting for involuntary movements of the laryngeal muscles leading to speech interruptions and/or a tight, strained voice

Spatial disorientation: the inability of a person to determine his true body position relative to the earth or his surroundings.

SPECT (Single Photon Emission Computed Tomography) scan: an imaging procedure done to assess metabolic function in a specific body part with the use of radioactive tracers

Speech therapy: Also known as speech language therapy, this involves the use of audio-visual aids and exercises for the treatment of language disorders and speech defects

SSRI (Selective serontonin reuptake inhibitor): medications used to treat anxiety and depression which acts by reducing serotonin re-absorption in the brain

Stimulant: medications that stimulate the central nervous system resulting to an elevated mood and increased alertness

Substantia nigra: a darkly pigmented area in the brainstem which contains dopamine-producing neurons; destruction of which is associated with Parkinson's disease

Sundowning: a manifestation of dementia which occurs late in the day into the night, characterized by agitation, increased confusion and disorientation

Sympathetic nervous system: a division of the autonomic nervous system which when activated results to an increased heart rate, blood vessel constriction and increased blood pressure

Synapse: junctions between neurons that functions for neurotransmitter transmission

Syncope: referred to as fainting, this involves a sudden, temporary loss of consciousness associated with insufficient blood and oxygen supply to the brain

Tactile hallucination: also known as somatic hallucination, this refers to hallucinations involving the sense of touch wherein a physical sensation localized within the body is falsely perceived by a person

Tau protein – normally found in the brain, abnormal synthesis leads to the formation of neurofibrillary tangles, which are involved in the development of neurodegenerative diseases such as Alzheimer's disease

Transient global amnesia -- sudden bouts of amnesia characterized by one's inability to recall recent events; usually lasting less than 24hrs

Tremor: Involuntary, rhythmical alteration in movement which can be attributed to stress, medications or neurological/metabolic diseases

Vascular dementia: most commonly seen in men, especially those with hypertension, this form of dementia affects small- and medium-sized cerebral vessels which undergo infarction producing multiple parenchymal lesions in the brain. Symptoms include language and memory impairment, confusion, agitation, personality and mood changes, and motor difficulties.

Visual hallucination: false sensory perception involving the sense of sight

Visuospatial dysfunction: inability to interpret geometric relationships manifested by patients with neurodegenerative disorders

Wanderer: persons who wander from place to place with no permanent addresses

Working memory: brain system that provides temporary storage of information necessary for short term use

References:

Burns A, Iliffe S. Alzheimer's disease. *BMJ*. 2009;338.

DeKosky ST, Kaufer DI, Hamilton RL, Wolk DA, Lopez OL. The dementias. In: Bradley WG, Daroff RB, Fenichel GM, Jankovic J, eds. *Bradley: Neurology in Clinical Practice*. 5th ed. Philadelphia, Pa: Butterworth-Heinemann Elsevier; 2008:chap 70.

Knopman DS. Alzheimer's disease and other dementias. In: Goldman L, Schafer AI, eds. *Cecil Medicine*. 24th ed. Philadelphia, Pa: Saunders Elsevier; 2011:chap 409.

Peterson RC. Clinical practice. Mild cognitive impairment. *N Engl J Med* 2011 Jun 9;364(23):2227-2234.

Qaseem A, et al., American College of Physicians/American Academy of Family Physicians Panel on Dementia. Current pharmacologic treatment of dementia: a clinical practice guideline from the American College of Physicians and the American Academy of Family Physicians. *Ann Intern Med* 2008 Mar 4;148(5):370-8.

From the Internet:
http://www.dvirsky.org.ua/psyedu/book/psychiatry.pdf
http://www.lewybodydementia.org/
http://www.ninds.nih.gov/disorders/dementiawithlewybodies/dementiawithlewybodies.htm
http://lbda.org/
http://www.lewybody.org/
http://www.mayoclinic.com/health/lewy-body-dementia/DS00795
http://www.caring.com/articles/dementia-with-lewy-bodies
http://brain.oxfordjournals.org/content/129/3/729.abstract
www.medicinenet.com
www.thefreedictionary.com
www.alzinfo.org/glossary/glossarywords.aspx
www.alz.org

Acknowledgments

Cover: Lisa F. Young | Fotolia.com

Dr. Andreas Becker | Wikimedia commons